My Twenty Year Journey

With PKD

In

The Dialysis World

My Twenty Year Journey With PKD In The Dialysis World

The History, My Family History, The Education

Of

Polycystic Kidney Disease

Managing Good Health on Hemodialysis and
Peritoneal Dialysis with the Renal Diet

A Second Invite into Glo's Renal Friendly Kitchen

Gloria Ann Jeff-Moore

To order additional copies of this book, contact:
Xlibris Corporation
1-888-795-4274
www.Xlibris.com
Orders@Xlibris.com
825093

CONTENTS

After sharing my first decade of dialysis experience, there were a number of readers, who wanted to know more about my second decade of dialysis history, in which I transitioned from a decade of hemo dialysis to peritoneal dialysis treatment, and I only hit the surface of my life with peritoneal dialysis, finally in this second book, you will learn more about my peritoneal dialysis copings in deeper detail.

There are bonuses included in this book such as the Standard Classification Chart for Blood Pressure, Chart Finders for foods (that indicate how much protein, potassium & phoshorus a particular food contains), so you can plan menus for a good renal diet, and of course mouth watering renal friendly recipes that are easy to prepare, and as a added bonus, you are invited to check out some more renal friendly recipes, along with some repeated recipes from my my first book, "My Renal Life" (I know it, I live it).

After sharing my dialysis experience and the knowledge that I have learned all these years, with fellow dialysis patients at my units, I was encouraged by techs and nurses at my unit, that I should share my experience with others out there, who maybe pending dialysis patients, as well as the fairly new dialysis patients, who could potentially benefit from my many years of experience. I know first hand, that this renal diet, can be quite a challenge, and very complexing at times, but I always say knowledge is key. I decided in the early 1990's, to educate myself as much as possible on the ends and outs of the renal diet, and even though I learned a great deal about the diet, applying it was not so easy. When you are raised a certain way on how to eat, and then all of a sudden, your current diet is not very healthy for this renal diet, then you have to do some compromising when it comes to this particular diet. The basic being, low sodium, low potassium and low phosphorus, and this was important for my renal diet, while on hem dialysis, but when I transitioned to PD, my renal diet changed somewhat, I was no longer having to monitor the amount of potassium I was consuming, because PD treatment, would eliminate my potassium in my body, so much more easily, and now I have a struggle, with eating enough potassium rich foods, that a potassium supplement, had to be prescribed for me.

EVERTHING YOU NEED TO KNOW ABOUT:

* *What's necessary to manage your health between Hemo dialysis treatment and everyday peritoneal dialysis Treatment*

* *What a renal diet consist of:*
* *The importance of controlling your blood pressure and if diabetic, controlling The blood sugar*
* *The significance of monthly lab testing*
* *Alternatives to having tasty, enjoyable food on a renal diet*
* *Keep the proteins up - to maintain healthy body weight*
* *The importance of exercising*

Dedicated
To
The Memory
Of

My father, the late Mr. Lionel Jeff, and my uncle, the late Mr. Leroy Calvin Jeff, both were an inspiration to me, because they both loved to write, and I feel that I was channeled by them both, to write about our family legacy of the polycystic kidney disease, to bring awareness to the most common genetic threatening disease out there, Polycystic Kidney Disease, (better referred to as PKD).

Acknowledgement

I want to once again thank my husband, Steven Moore, (20 year veteran of the Navy), for encouraging me to continue writing, and reminding me how therapeutic it has been for me, which has been very gratifying for me to share my experience that could potentially benefit other family members, as well as fellow dialysis patients, pending dialysis pts. and fairly new dialysis patients. I love him so much, for always accompanying me to my regular visits to my home dialysis unit.

My daughter, Tiffany Bianca M. Moore, now being an adult, she has given me so much inspiration through the years, and growing up to be a very beautiful young lady, with so much old wisdom, and how she has matured through all that I have had to endure with trials and tribulations of life on dialysis with PKD. And because what she has witness that I have gone through, all these years, and all that I have been through and have experienced, she wants to someday in the future become a vascular surgeon. I am so very proud of her.

My mom, Mrs. Rose Dell Jeff, even though we live a distance away from one another, she would always have some very spiritual and encouraging words of wisdom to share, I love her with all my heart, even though sometime we don't see eye to eye on some things. (LOL)

My cousin, (Titin), Irene Butler Celestine, whenever I needed a shoulder to cry on, she would only be a phone call away, and how she kept encouraging me to continue writing, to publish this second book, because I have so much more to share with the dialysis world.

My cousin, Carol Lynn Simpson Manciel, who always believe that I could be a great writer, and for all her help along the way, emotionally as well as financially, in promoting my first book.

My neprologist, Dr. Waseem Ahmad, in the last decade, has helped me to better understand this very unique life, and taking the time to always explain why this?, and why that?. I will never forget when he first came on the scene, after many months of making adjustments to certain medications, which wasn't showing any signs of improvement, and by the Grace of God, I was assigned a new neprologist (Dr. Waseem Ahmad), who immediately took over my case, and showed a great concern for my high level of parathyroid hormones, he didn't waste anytime scheduling surgery to have my glands removed immediately. He continues to be my neprologist this very day, and I thank God for bringing him into my life. It is always a delight to be in his presence.

Ray Moulin, for making my connection to Dr. Ahmad, very easy. Always available, when I call. Always on the ball, of getting any necessary paperwork completed, for one nature or another. And also helping in speeding up the process for my very important IVIG Procedure.

Jennifer Clary, Former Dietitian at Davita, Fairfield, who would always be straight up front about my lab values, and of course my diet. Chastising me, to eat more protein and potassium. She would call me once a month, to discuss my laboratory results, in which this helps me to get a better grasp on this very complex renal diet. I miss her so much.

Riquelen Ngumezi, LCSW, Davita, Fairfield, I haven't known her very long, but she has said on occasion, how very proud she is of me for sharing my dialysis experience in a published book to help others who could benefit from my many years of experience and knowledge. She also gave me the confidence to write a second book to share my second decade of life on dialysis with peritoneal dialysis.

Tyra LaChappelle, Former PD nurse, Davita, Fairfield, for being so precise and informative with the transitioning from hemo to peritoneal dialysis, although I didn't start my initial PD treatment at home, starting in the hospital was not planned, but her training helped a great deal in lessening my anxiety about doing treatment for the first time on my very own in the hospital setting, I miss her so very much.

My brother in law, David Moore, who also gave me the encouragement and confidence to write my second book, especially after all the endorsements that he express how brilliant, the writing of my first book, "My Renal Life" (I know it, I live it) was.

My two sisters, Alma Jean Bolden and Antoinette Jeff, who also are at present coping with the eff ects of Polycystic Kidney Disease, and have in the last few years started Dialysis, as treatment to further sustain their lives, (Antoinette in 2007, and Alma, in early 2010), they are both currently on the waiting list for a kidney transplant.

My niece, April LaMont, also affected by PKD, I will never forget the very humble conversation we had, when I was on a vacation visit to her parents home in Connecticut, back in the fall of 2003, she ask me if she will have to do this treatment, but through the blessing of her father, Robert LaMont, she received her dads kidney in 2007, with great success and she also became a 2010 high school graduate, and will be entering college in the Fall, I am so very proud of her, she is today living a very normal young adult life.

Introduction

The fortunate fact that renal failure is becoming more and more prevalent in today's society, and of course, the fact that I have witness in the last decade, there are more younger adults, as well as older teens developing end stage renal disease, (from one nature or another), and most importantly, those individuals that have a history of diabetes and/or high blood pressure, (two of the main causes, of the development of chronic kidney disease). Because of our aging population, and more and more baby boomers are surviving these days, kidney disease (failure) is affecting more people today than ever before. Today more people suffer from diabetes, high blood pressure, heart disease and obesity. Many diseases have the potential to damage kidneys, impairing their ability to filter waste effectively and ultimately produces a life-threatening situation. The lack of education about the kidneys and how important it is to our health in general, is the main reason why the kidneys can go unnoticed with the possibility of early stages of chronic kidney disease, and what can happen when they began to fail. The good thing is that they have developed a way to help in monitoring the stages of chronic kidney disease (meaning the kidney function), and seeking early testing for the early stages of chronic kidney disease, could be so beneficial, because preventive measures can be taken early on, to help in prolonging or even in some cases can possibly reverse the progression of chronic kidney disease. In the last few years, our San Francisco Chapter of the PKD Foundation, has been vigorously bringing awareness of chronic kidney disease, and to continue urging individuals to go get tested for the early stages of CKD, especially those that are aware of a family history of PKD, and of course the two main causes of CKD, (diabetes and/or high blood pressure). CKD has been identified as a silent but deadly multiplier of other major chronic kidney diseases, such as diabetes and/or high blood pressure, lupus, glumerulonephritis, FSGS, PKD, and other natures such as illness, injury, and prolonged medication regiment of some kind. I have a great deal to share in this second book of life with PKD and dialysis, but this time, with peritoneal dialysis, in which I am in my 10th year of PD treatment. I have also put it into my mind, that after coping with PKD for so long with the help of the blessing of the creation of dialysis as my life sustain treatment, I would learn as much as I can about PKD, which seems to still until this very day, have a stigma of mystery attached to it. Not learning much from my dad or previous family members, who could never tell me much about the disease, I felt it was time for me to research PKD, and find out as much as I can, to get a better understanding of when this disease was first introduced in my family history, and how it could have occurred. I would also like to share my father's copings with PKD and dialysis way back in the early 1970's. Through my research, I will share some of what I have discovered about my Grandmother, Madea, what she had to cope with, with her saga with poly cystic kidney disease (in which they didn't know what exactly caused her kidney failure). I will also share my humble beginning of my saga with PKD and dialysis. You will also get a peek into my dialysis life with peritoneal dialysis, and how I managed vs. hemo dialysis. And last but not least, I invite my readers into this second edition, into Glo's Renal Friendly Kitchen. Now, I know most of you readers may already know how important normal functioning kidneys are to the body, and what exactly does the kidneys do, but if you don't know, I would like to include this knowledge, so you can get a better understanding of why it is so important to take care of what health issue, to keep the kidneys healthy, a little education about the kidneys is in order. Check out these important facts.

Those Important Organs - The Kidneys

The Kidneys are two of your most important organs. They perform vital functions such as: waste removal, blood filtering and blood pressure regulating. When the kidneys are healthy - they maintain the body's internal equilibrium of water and minerals (sodium, potassium, chloride, calcium, phosphorus, and magnesium sulfate). Kidneys also remove from the blood, the daily metabolic load of fixed hydrogen ions. Kidneys can become so damaged by disease or injury, that they no longer clean waste products from the blood, which this can lead to Acute Kidney Failure - which is a sudden usually short-term loss of kidney function, but another serious kidney failure called End Stage Renal Disease, could result from the progression of chronic kidney disease. End Stage Renal Disease is a permanent, and irreversible damage to both kidneys, which the most common causes of ESRD is diabetes and/or high blood pressure. Diabetes can damage blood vessels in the kidneys and is one of the primary causes of kidney disease, but there are others such as high blood pressure, lupus, glomerulonephritis, and the inherited kidney disease called poly cystic kidney disease, in which I have, and PKD is the main topic of this book. When chronic kidney disease results into end stage renal disease, dialysis or the blessing of a transplant, becomes absolutely necessary for continued survival. As I have mentioned in my first book "My Renal Life" (I know it, I live it), it is a fact that dialysis isn't a cure for failing kidneys, however, dialysis treatment does clean your blood and removes excessive fluid, somewhat like normal kidneys do, but it also removes needed minerals that your body needs, and it doesn't balance the calcium and phosphorus in your body. Dialysis does replace some of these functions through diffusion (waste removal) and ultra filtration (fluid removal). Dialysis is a life saving treatment for people who have developed end stage renal disease. I know that all this may sound discouraging, and may give you some uncertainties of living on dialysis, but I am here to tell you, you can live a long, and productive life with dialysis as a part of it. There are patients like myself, who are living a very long and productive life with dialysis, this very day. For me, living this long on dialysis, it has become second nature to me, and yes, I thought the very same way in the beginning, that I didn't know if I could live my life this way for very long, and I proved my own self wrong, you can say I ate my own words (so to speak). Twenty years and still going strong. Now, lets talk about the main topic of this book - Polycystic Kidney Disease, better known in the dialysis world as PKD. I have mentioned that I have the Poly cystic Kidney Disease, and you may be curious as to what exactly is the Poly cystic Kidney Disease, well, read on, because the next chapter of this book, I will share with you, what actually is PKD.

What is The Polycystic Kidney Disease

Poly cystic Kidney Disease, also referred to as PKD, are fluid filled sacs in the kidney, (called cysts), but having some cysts is harmless, but having poly (meaning many) cystic kidney disease may cause the kidneys to become abnormally large. This condition is inherited.

Renal cyst begin forming in ureter and increase in size and numbers throughout the affected persons lifetime resulting in ESRD. Although PKD is the most common genetic threatening disease, (more common than sickle cell anemia, cystic fibrosis, muscular dystrophy, and down syndrome combined), there is a stigma of mystery attached to PKD, especially where my family history is concerned. I have traced it back (as I stated previously in the introduction of this book) as far back as my Grandma Madea, who was suffering with it back in the late 1940's, and at that time there wasn't any mention of a name for this disease, that my Grandma had, (more about my Grandma Madea's poly cystic kidney disease saga is included in the chapter titled - My Family History).

What was discovered is that the faulty gene can disable the kidney with 100's of cyst, which fill with fluid and can be as large as an egg or some can be even larger. Cyst can crowd out cells and make the kidneys began to fail, if this happens the cyst can swell even more.

It was discovered that there are two types of PKD, one being Autosomal Dominant and other Autosomal Recessive PKD.

Autosomal Dominant - referred to as ADPKD - if one parent has the disease, there is a 50% chance that the disease will pass to a child. At least one parent must have the disease for a child to inherit it. Either the mother or father can pass it along, but new mutations may account for ¼ of new cases. In some rare cases, the cause of ADPKD occurs spontaneously in the child soon after conception. In these cases, the parent are not the source of this disease.

Autosomal Recessive PKD - referred to as ARPKD - Is caused by a particular genetic flow that is different from the genetic flow that causes ARPKD.

ADPKD - Parents who do not have the disease can have a child with the disease, if both parents carry the abnormal gene and both pass the gene to their baby. The chances of this happening (when both parents carry the abnormal gene), is one in four. If only one parent carries the abnormal gene, the baby cannot get the disease. I know this disease sounds very complicated, doesn't it? Well, at least there is more that is known about PKD today, than there was many decades ago. There are some people that I have come across in my dialysis journey, that don't even know who they may have inherited PKD from, and that is truly unfortunate, because at least I do know who I inherited the disease from, but many generations of my family, never knew who they could have inherited the disease from, especially from the research that I have discovered about my family history of the disease. So many unanswered questions, but I have learned through the years, a little about PKD, and how it may have been introduced in my family gene pool.

Now, that I have shared a little education about PKD, let's talk about possible first signs and symptoms of PKD - as indicated on the following page

Possible First Signs and Symptoms of PKD

Note: These signs and symptoms are very important towards being tested for the possible early stage of Chronic Kidney Disease - (You will learn more about the benefits of early testing of chronic kidney disease)

Blood in urine - which may come and go, this is due to one or more cyst bleeding from time to time

Protein in urine

Pain over one or both kidneys. This is due to the enlarged kidneys.

Kidney stones (can occur in people with ADPKD). Symptoms of kidney stones can range from no symptoms at all to very severe pain, if a stone becomes blocked in the ureter.

What is Kidney Stones?

They are hard deposits that form in the kidneys, which can block drainage. They may be caused by excess calcium in the urine.

Risk factors for the possibility of the development of kidney stones is - Dehydration, prolong use of alcohol, excess vitamin D, and/or a family history of kidney stones.

Abdominal pain and/or swollen abdomen

High Blood Pressure

Recurring kidney infections

Note: These symptoms may alert a doctor to investigate further and diagnose ADPKD, and when that is the diagnosed result, then further testing for possible development of CKD could be present. If diagnosed with CKD, what stage is it at., and hopefully the test show that it is in the early stages of CKD, and then preventive measures can be taken early on, to prolong or even reverse the progression of CKD., but in some cases with PKD, it is inevitable that CKD, could result into end stage renal disease (Stage 5)., and then the end result of that, is that dialysis or the blessing of a transplant, becomes absolutely necessary to sustain the renal patients life. Usually an ultrasound scan of the kidneys is done, and then a urine test to check for blood and protein in the urine. Blood test are primarily done to check on the function of the kidneys. Further testing is also done with a CT Scan and MRI Scan.

Statistics of Poly cystic Kidney Disease

Statistics show that there are over 600,000 individuals that have been diagnosed with PKD in the United States, and 12.5 million worldwide, and there are potential others out there, that haven't as of yet, been diagnosed, so in my opinion, if you have knowledge of a family history of PKD, I strongly urge individuals out there to go get tested for the possibility of PKD, and of course, if diagnosed with PKD, further finding out what stage of CKD are they in, so that preventive measures can be taken early on, in prolonging the onset of the development of End Stage Renal Disease (Stage 5), and we know the end result of that, is a form of dialysis or the blessing of a kidney, becomes absolutely necessary to sustain their lives. PKD is one of the most common genetic threatening diseases out there, more common than sickle cell anemia, cystic fibrosis, muscular dystrophy, and down syndrome combined, but yet this very day, there is a stigma of mystery attached to this disease, I can't stress this enough. When I first started dialysis, some two decades ago, I was surprised to find there were actual veteran dialysis patients, that haven't even heard of PKD, and of course, even dialysis patients with PKD, truly didn't know much about PKD, for that matter. I myself, only know what I have learned, since starting dialysis treatment, but through these years that I have been on dialysis, I decided to do some research on what exactly is PKD, then after my findings, I decided to research my family history of PKD, and yes, I found out some very interesting facts about my family, and you will discovered in a later chapter, a little about my findings.

GFR Facts

GFR - which stands for Glomerular Filtration Rate - This is the best test to measure your level of kidney function and determine your stage of kidney disease. The doctor can calculate it from the results of your blood creatinine test, your age, race, gender and nature of the development of CKD. The earlier the disease is detected, the better the chance of slowing or stopping its progression. Here is a little education to share with you, on how the GFR works to help those who are being monitored in stages of CKD.

Stages of Chronic Kidney Disease (CKD):

Stage 1 - 90% kidney function
Diagnose and try to reverse the cause of decreased kidney function - GFR - 130
Stage 2 - 60-89% kidney function
Try to stem the progression of CKD - GFR - 90
Stage 3 - 30-59% kidney function
Try to continue to stem the progression of CKD - GFR - 60

Stage 4 - 15-29% kidney function
Explore dialysis/transplantation - GFR - 30
Stage 5 - less than 15% kidney function
Dialysis/transplant becomes absolutely necessary for continued survival - GFR - 15-0

Note: Renal Patient with increased kidney function, should avoid taking any kind of pain medication, because it has the potential to make the kidney disease worse. Always check with your health care provider, before taking any medicine, and by all means, if you are a smoker, and you are diagnosed with the early stages of CKD, quit smoking, because smoking not only increases the risk of kidney disease, but it also contributes to deaths from strokes and heart attacks in people with CKD.

A GFR of 90 or above is considered normal functioning kidneys, moderate decrease in GFR of (30-59), at this stage of CKD, hormones and minerals can be thrown out of balance, leading to anemia and weak bones. Your health care provider can help in preventing or treat this complication with medicines and advice about food choices. Severe reduction of GFR (15 to 29), the treatment should continue with the treatment for complications of CKD and keep educating themselves as much as possible about the treatments of kidney failure. And of course once the patients GFR is less than 15, they are in end stage renal disease (Stage 5), and a form of dialysis or transplantation because necessary to sustain their lives.

My Introduction to the Dialysis World

Pre-dialysis, when I was first diagnosed with End Stage Renal Disease (ESRD), I wasn't being monitored in stages of chronic kidney disease with the creation of GFR, I was only told that I had developed ESRD, and needed hemo dialysis real soon., he didn't even give me a choice of choosing hemo or PD. And besides for that matter, he didn't even mention peritoneal dialysis (PD) at all., I didn't even know that this form of dialysis was in existence. (I share later on in the book, about my first discovery of when I exactly had knowledge of Peritoneal Dialysis), I had the surgery for the placement of an access, and it was soon discovered that I wasn't a candidate for a fistula, which is the best access to have for hemo, because of the potentially long lifespan of having a fistula, and there is less risk of developing an infection, verses having a graft, which has more of a risk of developing an infection, and of course, clotting issues. I had to have what they called an AV Graft, (because I had very small veins), so a graft had to be surgically put in place. This is a fairly harmless surgical procedure, where my artery was connected to a vein, using a synthetic tube or graft, implanted under the skin in my arm. The graft became an artificial vein that can be used repeatedly for needle placement and blood access during hemo dialysis. It matured in about three to four weeks, unlike if I had a fistula, which takes about six to eight weeks to heal and mature for usage. Back in 1990, when I had the graft surgically place, I was admitted over night, but all this has changed in the last decade and a half, patients today usually can go home several hours after the surgery. What I do remember about this surgical procedure, is that my arm felt like it was made of rubber, when I touched it in the recovery room, and that I had no control over my arm, which they told me, to not move it around at all and this feeling that I felt when I touched my arm, was because my arm was administered IV meds to put my arm to sleep, so to speak, for the surgical procedure. Now before I get deeper into this particular topic, let me first, apologize to those readers that purchased my first book, I know you may or may not be aware that the spelling of graft, was misspelled, (graph, to be exact), well I was aware of this, but it was too late or shall I say too expensive to make those changes, and again I apologize for the misspelled word, as this was my first attempt at self-publishing, I will do my best to make sure that I don't have any misspelled words in this book. Now, back to my Graft saga, Like I said, I was admitted to a patient room, and my vitals were taken several times during the night. I know what I didn't have, was an appetite, so they changed my diet to a liquid type diet for that day, you know the usual, consisting of chicken broth, jello and apple sauce. The next morning, I regain my appetite, and was able to eat a full breakfast. Later on that day, I was discharged from the hospital, and by this time, my arm was feeling like a arm should feel normally. I was home for about a month, going through the healing process of the Graft. It was the fourth week, and I was beginning to experience a great deal of swelling in my feet, and then vomiting more and more, even the pink stuff kept coming up, nothing was no longer staying down. Just about everything that I would consume in my diet, I would throw up, I also was experiencing very frequent urinating, which at times, I would have those frequent miss the toilet accidents, you know, (can't get my pants off, before I get on the toilet, but I soon remedied that situation, I started wearing skirts and dresses, so I can get to my underwear much quicker, (lol) I want to share with you my true wakeup call, that I know it was time to start hemo dialysis as soon as possible, (I had just gotten off the bart (transportation service that I would take from San Francisco to the East Bay) from work, I got off the bart and walked to the parking lot to my car, and drove over to the daycare to pick up my toddler daughter, a routine that I did every day of the week, and of course, I picked my daughter up, and was on my way home, and as soon as I got into the underground garage of my apartment building, I got that darn urge, (you know), I had to pissed so bad, I was practically breaking my neck to get up to my apartment, where I would usually wait for the elevator, I dashed up the back stairs, which would get me up to my apartment on the second floor much quicker, (and of course, time was not on my side). I got to the front door of my apartment, and for some strange reason, I was finding it difficult to get the key to work, I guest it was because I was panicking, because boy I sure didn't want to have another one of those accident, (you know where I couldn't hold it long enough to get to the toilet), and as I was struggling to get the key in the keyhole, my neighbor Shirley, across the hall, was looking out her window, and noticed that I was taking way too long to get inside my apartment, and she immediately ask, Gloria, are you having difficulty with your key, but before I could say anything, my daughter, yells out, "Mommy got to pee real bad", it could have been an hilarious moment, but I was the victim, and I know if I would have allowed myself to laugh, I know I would have piss on myself, so I just smiled at the neighbor, and finally I got the door open, but I wasn't too disappointed this time, because remember, I told you, I started wearing nothing but skirts and dresses, so hallelujah! I made it to the toilet, without leaking a drop on myself, this wasn't my true wakeup call, I could remember as though it happened yesterday, I was employed at the University of San Francisco, as the department secretary in the College of Business, and Professor Singleton (one of thirty professors, that I assist with secretarial duties), hands me a document to fax to Uruguary, and a exam and the key to be typed for his midterm exam. I immediately sent the fax, and continued by typing the key for the exam, but at the time, when Professor Singleton requested these items to be done, it was 12:45, and I only did about a third of the key, and then it was 1:00 p.m. , and it was time for my lunch break, so I immediately went over to the student lodge, because it was also time for my favorite soap, "One Life to Live", and God knows I didn't want to miss this episode, because it happen to be the episode, about Lantano Mountain, and that underground city called Eternal, I got to the student lodge, just in time, and got comfortable, with my made at home lunch, (so I didn't have to lose any time to buy any lunch), as I was getting into the soap, Guess What! I got that darn urge again, and of course, I was stubborn about leaving right then and there, to relieve myself, so I decided that as soon as the commercial started, I would dash around the corner to the restroom, well I went inside the restroom, and went straight into the stall, (that was facing the door), and didn't have a accident, Thank God! I was very pleased about this, but as I was washing my hands, I happened to look in the mirror, and noticed that there was this long steel object against the wall behind me, and then I took a very quick turn to look around the restroom, and didn't notice a tampon dispenser of any kind, that is when I immediately realized that I was indeed in the Men's restroom, well I was lucky no one was in the restroom at the time, so I quickly tried to make my escape from the restroom, as promptly as I could, but guess who walks in, yes I'm sure you guessed it, professor Singleton, and he promptly sees me, and ask me, if I sent the fax, and I answered, and was still trying to get out of that restroom, but he kept talking, and continued by asking me, did I complete the exam and key for his midterm, and at that moment, it darned on me, that he must have forgotten where he was, better yet, why in the hell was I in the Men's restroom. I looked at him with embarrassment, and said frantically,

"I still haven't finished the key and I got to get out of here, finally I got out of the restroom, and back to the student lodge, but by that time, I couldn't focus on the show, because all I could think about was that little embarrassing incident in the Men's restroom. After having this very embarrassing moment, I then alerted this to my neprologist, (well not the part about the restroom ordeal, but the vomiting up everything that I consumed), and he informed me that I needed to start hemo treatment right away, then after making that call, Professor Singleton walks in, and I immediately ask him, Did he realized that I was in the Men's restroom, and he kinda looked at me sort of crossed like, and I said, is it that you are all business, all the time, and anywhere. Well, he was finally in the land of the living, and apologized to me, for that little situation. Previously weeks before having the surgery for my Graft, I visited the unit that would one day soon become my home unit. The pre-dialysis and initial day of hemo treatment was shared in my first published book, "My Renal Life" (I know it, I live it)., published back in February of 2009., under the topic "Adjusting to the Dialysis World", but I will repeat this segment in this book. However, after the initial treatment, and about a few weeks later, I was experiencing these sides effects that the "The Renal Divas", had discuss previously over one of our Friday roundtable chatting discussions. You will learn about the renal divas in the chapter titled - . "My Family History of Poly cystic Kidney Disease".

A month after my initial start of hemo dialysis, I had my first experience with my blood pressure plummeting, and it felt as though I was dying. I also experienced this cramping of the body, (in which the renal divas chatted about during one of our many Friday chats over lunch). These cramps and drastically dropping b/p episodes went on frequently. About ten months into hemo dialysis, I came into the unit, and it was discovered by the dialysis tech, that my Graft had clotted. When this happened, I obviously couldn't have hemo treatment, and my neprologist, (who was most of the time in his office, in the very same building that I was having treatment), was informed of this, and he immediately schedule me for emergency surgery to declot my Graft, which was a pretty mild surgical procedure. At this time, I still wasn't discharged the same day back then, but now they do discharge a patient, after having their Graft declotted. I actually came back to the unit, with a subclavian (catherer), for several weeks. I returned to have my hemo treatment in one of their isolation rooms, (in which hemophiliacs are normally having treatment), I guess they thought it was more safer and sanitary to have subclavian used for treatment in this room. What I didn't like about having treatment this way for the first time, is the fact that the treatment didn't go as smoothly, like my actual graft usually does, and it is not so comfortable and relaxing to dialyze from a catherer, because I was told to not move around much, and I was reclined so far back in the dialyzing chair, that it was very uncomfortable. Also while having this subclavian, (which was placed in my chest), there is a increased risk of getting it infected, and I had to be very careful while dialyzing this way. My dialyzing time with this catherer was for three and half hours, compared to when my graft is used, which normally is scheduled for two and half hours. Through this ten year journey in the hemo dialysis world, I had numerous catheters placed in my neck, chest and groin. The advantage to having a catherer for dialyzing is, that there is no needling required. Finally, after a month of this catheterization method of dialyzing, my catherer was removed in the unit by the unit nurse, and it was time to resume using my graft again. So, on with the three days a week dialyzing ritual (M,W,F). Having an AV Graft, there are risk of the development of low blood flow, in which I developed several times during my 10 year run with hemo dialysis. This low blood flow that I developed with my Graft, was an indication of clotting and the narrowing of the access. Through a echocardiogram, that was ordered by my cardiologist, the results showed a problem with my heart, because it was starting to work harder, so this required me to have a procedure called an angiography, and this was then ordered by my cardiologist. This procedure involves taking x-ray pictures of my blood vessels. These x-rays can show the location and severity of blockages in my vessels. The scenarios that surround having this procedure, is pretty harmless. After having my vitals checked, I was then instructed to disrobe completely, I was then taken to the cath lab, where the angiography was being done, and placed on a x-ray table, and I was then given a sedative to help me to relax, because I was having a great deal of anxiety, and I had never had a procedure of such before, so I didn't quite know what to expect. After the sedative was administered, my skin in the area of the insertion site was marked and very thoroughly cleanse, and then the insertion site was numbed (my left groin to be exact), a sheath was inserted into my artery in the groin, the sheath remained in place during the entire procedure. During this phase of the cath procedure, the blood vessels don't have no pain nerves, so I didn't really feel any phase of this procedure. After this procedure was completed, and the results were looked at by the doctor, he then discussed the results with me, remember I am awake during these proceedings, I was only administered IV meds to relax me, so I was fully alert. I was then told by the doctor, that I would have an angioplasty, to improve my blood flow of my access. The end result was to have balloon angioplasty, and I was told what will transpire during this mild procedure, it was done using a catherer, which was done right after the angiography procedure. The surgeon used the catherer to insert a special balloon into the artery. The balloon was then inflated and deflated a few times to open the artery. It was followed by the placement of a stent. Stenting - is a wire mesh that was inserted into my artery to hold it open. It was left permanently in my artery. I was also informed that I was given a drug-eluting stent. I'm always curious about everything to do with any procedure that I am to undergo, so I then asked, what was a drug-eluting stent? , and the surgeon informed me that it is a stent that releases medication over time to help in keeping scar tissue from forming as my artery is healing. Because after the catheterization procedure was done, and the results showed that I needed an angioplasty procedure, I wasn't allowed to go home, I was then admitted to a room. I was closely monitored, my pulse, blood pressure and temp was checked very often. My IV line was still in place, and another electrocardiogram was done to access the condition of my blood flow. I was told to lie very still during the night, my groin site was check once again by the nurse, as well as the doctor, to make sure there was no indication of any bleeding from the site, and everything checked out fine, and I was allowed to be discharged. Since my insertion site was in the groin, I was given instructions by the nurse to take a sponge bath for a few days, and no swimming or soaking in a tub of water. I was also told to not do any lifting of anything over ten pounds for at least three days. I had to also avoid strenuous activities for about a week. Also no driving was included in this restriction, and of course no sexual activities (ha!!ha!). I was OK with that, but I don't think my husband was too enthuse with this particular restriction (lol). I had a follow up with my cardiologist. She prescribed medication for my condition, and also strongly suggested I can do regular exercise to help in keeping my heart healthy. Of course, I have never been a smoker, so that wasn't an issue with me, to stop smoking. Going through the motion of artery problems with my AV Graft access, I began to have issues with edema. This truly became apparent, when I had my first cadaver kidney transplant. During the time when I had my first transplant, I had to have some further hemo dialysis treatment, but my graft clotted, and they decided to have a subclavian surgically place on the left side of my neck, but it was a very blotched up surgery to have it put in place. Because of the subclavian swelling up so severely, (when I returned to hemo after losing the transplanted kidney after four months with a major rejection), I immediately started having issues with severe swelling of my body. The severity of the edema, prompted my neprologist to have an additional Graft put in place, because he believed it would relieve the swelling from happening, because of my current Graft edema issues, this was not the solution, because the swelling continued and it got so severe, that most times, I truly didn't look like myself in appearance, the swelling truly affected my face so badly, that I could hardly see. Other parts of my body was effected, especially the left side of my body. My legs and feet were another issue, that I had to result to wearing nothing but clogs and slip on shoes, well anyway, it was in my favor during this time, because slip-ons and clogs were in style as a footwear fashion statement, and I had invested in just about every style imaginable. I shared this little tidbit, just in case, there was other fellow dialysis pts, who have issues with serious edema issues with their feet expanding. In my first book, "My Renal Life", (I know it, I live it), I shared the first decade of my life with my journey in the hemo dialysis world, but I didn't get very detailed in my first book about my coping with peritoneal dialysis treatment, in which many of my readers wanted to know more about my ten year hemo dialysis experience and mostly importantly, what transpired with my AV Graft, this very much prompt me to share more deeply my experience with hemo dialysis. Now, after a ten year run with hemo dialysis, and numerous AV Grafts and repairs of angioplasties and temporary catherer, my fourth and last Graft issues became so very serious, that I had an episode at home, where my Leg graft, (which happen to be placed in the upper part of my left thigh), burst in the shower, and it was so out of control, if you would have been there, you would've thought that I had struck oil or something, blood was shooting straight in the air, and splattered all over the bathroom, and my bedroom, where I was trying to call for help from any family member. Of course, the paramedics were summoned, and they attempted to bring the bleeding under control. I won't repeat the episode in full detail, because it was thoroughly detailed in my first book. So, on with what happened after repairs to my graft, which wasn't properly repaired, and when I returned to hemo treatment the following day, a major problem arosed, because of a dialysis tech not listening to the instructions that were given to me by the vascular surgeon, (who did emergency surgery to repair my graft). I was told by the surgeon, to not let the tech bring the blood flow to no more than 250 to start, and gradually raise the pressure, but this tech didn't pay any attention to my request, and put the blood flow to the normal pressure, as if I had a perfectly functioning graft, she programmed it for the 350, and that was a major mistake, which caused great trauma and pain at the graft site. I felt this pain all the way up to my left side of my buttock (rump). I was immediately transported by ambulance to the hospital. I had the surgery, but it was evident that I wouldn't be able to use this graft anymore, and because of all the problems with grafts and repairs, and catheters in the upper part of my body, which caused very severe swelling of my body, I had to resort to having a catheter placed in the groin on the right side. I was also told that this was temporary, because I had no other alternative but to transition from hemo to peritoneal dialysis treatment. Going through the motions of transitioning to PD from hemo, having hemo treatment first and then going to the PD department to begin my training for PD treatment, this went on for about a month, but during this time, the surgery that I had when I had the leg graft episode, didn't heal properly, because during the time when I had the surgery procedure, a Jackson Pratt, (it was a tube with a plastic bag like substance attached to the tube), which was placed in my leg to help with the draining of the inflammation (better refer to as pus), this would develop, as the wound was healing, but it didn't collect in the Jackson Pratt, like it was suppose to, it was constantly collecting in my leg, where the graft was located. My vascular surgeon, checked the Jackson Pratt device, during the first follow up visit and he noticed that the pus wasn't collecting in this device, he promptly ask did I have any breakfast, before coming to see him, and I informed him that I didn't, I didn't always eat breakfast every morning, but it was a fortunate thing, that I didn't eat anything this very morning. My surgeon was pleased with this, because he said I needed emergency surgery to relieve this inflammation in my leg, immediately. This went on for several weeks, (getting drained three times), before the decision was made after the surgeon carefully examined my leg, he finally decided to go through my foot to finally get rid of this problem with my leg, and by this time, it was time to take the temporary catheter from my groin, and I was to start peritoneal dialysis. Although I had very good training from my PD nurse, Tyra, who was very thorough and precise with the training that I did grasped from the few weeks of training, it helped a great deal with the process of starting my initial treatment, while hospitalized, which I soon discovered that the nurses were apparently a little rusty with the PD procedure, I had to practically do the PD exchanges on my own. I did however, draw a diagram of the ultra bag, that was used to do the PD exchanges, and I happened to have the pad, that I took notes, while training at the unit for my transition to PD from Hemo. I remembered all of the important facts about doing the exchanges as safely and secured as possible, to prevent the development of peritonitis, (an infection that could occur with PD treatment), Tyra, (unit PD nurse), stress this constantly through the training, and I commend her, because I truly benefited from her expert PD training.

A caution to all AV Graft patients from Glo (a veteran AV Graft patient)

I decided to include my plight with my graft access, because there maybe other fellow dialysis pts, who have chosen hemo dialysis, as their means of treatment, and they may also have the very same issues as I do, (very small veins), and this meant that I had to have an AV Graft surgically placed, instead of a AV Fistula, (which is so much better to have). What I am trying to stress, is if a patient doesn't have no alternative, but to have AV Graft, and of course, if it starts to give them some of the health issues, that I have experienced in the past, it is OK to have a second Graft, but if that begins to fail, please, and trust me, don't considerate having another Graft, because these Graft have the potential to be very taxing on the body, to the point that other health issues can arise. I think in my opinion, the edema was the reason why I developed congestive heart failure, (the techs and nurses at the unit, not succeeding in getting me to my targeted dry weight, and because of my severe edema, the nurses and techs at the unit, had the most difficult time, trying to figure out, what was edema and what appeared to be excessive fluid, because I was coming in so severely swollen, I know this was a trauma to my heart, which may have caused my development of congestive heart failure, which usually that happens, when there is an excessive amount of fluid on board, which can flood the lungs, and caused the heart to enlarge, and that is what actually happened to me. Never being able to calculate the right amount of fluid to remove, was very frustrating for the techs at the unit, but they did their best, to try to get me to my dry weight, it was truly a guessing game, when it came to how much was fluid and how much was edema, but by the grace of god, everything worked out, although it was very trying for me, because I developed breathing difficulty, because of all this, even when I would sleep I had to sleep on top of three or four pillows, to even get a good night of sleep.

Also, sharing my pre-dialysis experience, can give you a better understanding of how advanced the dialysis world has become, today individuals, are encouraged to get tested for the early stages of chronic kidney disease, (especially those that have a family history of a particular kidney disease, diabetes and/or high blood pressure). If diagnosed in the early stages, they will not have to go through what I went through pre-dialysis, (you know, those frequent miss the toilet accidents), just uncontrollable pissing (excuse my French). Since GFR has come into play, a renal patient can be monitored more closely, and preventive measures can be taken earlier on, in prolonging the onset of the development of end stage renal disease, and in some cases, chronic kidney disease, can be reversed from the progression to end stage renal disease, but don't fret! If your CKD does develop into ESRD, don't think it is the end of the world for you, because you can live productively with dialysis, no matter how long it takes to receive the blessing of a kidney, whether it be living or a cadaver.

So, AV Graft patients, getting one or two grafts is ok, but when that second one fails, please don't consider getting a third one, because trust me, your veins will soon become less friendly to you. I know considering a transition to PD, could be devastating to you, especially if you have gotten real comfortable with hemo dialysis. I can protest to this, because when I was told that after having my fourth graft, (which was placed in my left upper thigh), that I would have no other alternative, but to do peritoneal dialysis, as my means of continued dialysis treatment, I had no other choice, but to accept this, but I must admit I didn't agree to it right away, I was being very stubborn about PD, because of what I was hearing about it, I truly didn't want my stomach invaded for this particular dialysis treatment, and after two weeks of contemplating, and most importantly, reflecting on my ten year journey with hemo dialysis, all that I have endured - the graft issues, the renal diet, the development of congestive heart failure, the edema saga, a clot lurking in my body, four bleeding stomach ulcers, and the numerous surgeries for one health issue or another, yes it was time, to decide to transition to PD, because I had gone through so much, my body had had enough invasion of trauma, and it needed a break. Now, today I am in my 10th year of PD, and I don't regret ever making this change, it has been so much better for me, less hospital stays, and of course, my body isn't getting abused so much now. Now, don't get me wrong, there are things that I missed about hemo, and I truly realized early on, that PD was far less taxing on my body. For instance, on hemo, I could be administered certain meds during my hemo treatment, and that of course, bares no pain, whereas with PD, some meds had to be administered by needling, and there are some that I have to take orally with PD, - such as: say for instance, if I needed more iron, on hemo I could have it administered through the tubing, during the hemo treatment, and EPO, (Epogen), which is administered during hemo treatment, but of course, the EPO has to be given in a shot form, when on PD. Now, of course, PD requires needling for EPO, whereas hemo doesn't require any needling of any kind. PD is a pretty harmless form of dialysis treatment. The one thing that is a risk with PD, is the fact, that a patient, especially someone who is small frame, like myself, may develop a umbilical hernia, in which I developed in my six year of PD, and I have been living with this hernia, for almost four years now, and due to all the access problems that I have, while on hemo, my nephrologist agreed that it wasn't a good idea for me to have to go back to hemo temporarily, because the only place I could have a catherer was in my groin, and that is very taxing on me, with the stigma of restrictions attached to it. I was told that I had an existing hernia, during a temporary transition back to hemo, because of a development of a fungus, (which the PD catherer had to be taken completely out). However, I wasn't aware of any hernia, that I had, (no visible indication of such), but I was told by the vascular surgeon that I had a existing hernia, (which wasn't visible to me at all), so I was a little bit surprised to know this, but after having this double deal, to put my PD catherer back in and also repair this so called hernia, that I had, After about six months after I was back on the PD, I sure enough, developed a hernia, that was quite visible. My nephrologist, right then and there decided after how taxing it was for me, when I returned to hemo temporarily, that if I don't have any discomfort or pain, with having this hernia, he won't suggest having the hernia repaired). Now, I am in my fourth year of having this hernia, and I haven't had any pain or discomfort for that matter, but what I do have, is an extra protruding stomach, besides the slightly protruding stomach from the solution that I have to dwell in my body. Since then, I have been filling less solution in my peritoneum, (to keep less pressure on the existing hernia), but I have been doing fine with this. Although this kind of thing happened to me, it doesn't necessary mean it will happen to you, but be wise, all you small frame patients, there is a potential to develop a hernia from PD treatment.

Adjusting to the Dialysis World

When I was first diagnose with End Stage Renal Disease (ESRD) - (meaning Kidney Failure), I knew this meant that I would have to make one of the most important changes of my life. My health became a priority, second in line to my toddler daughter, who I was raising as a single parent. I began to live a very organized life, once dialysis became a part of it. Being spontaneous was no longer a part of the plan. Three days a week I spent an excessive amount of my life at a dialysis unit, which I soon referred to as my second home. Five years had passed after giving birth to my premature daughter, due to the development of preclampsia (is a condition, where the placenta can be prevented from getting enough blood), and I was hospitalized for the second time with a very severe kidney infection, which resulted to my kidney failure becoming an immediate serious matter. I had the surgical procedure to have an access inserted in my arm at that time for dialysis treatment. Mind you, I was one of the lucky ones, because I found out that some individuals weren't as fortunate as I was to have a waiting period and time to reflect on the life without dialysis for a little while longer. I thank God for that, and I treasured my last days without dialysis to the utmost. I was discharged after a week of antibiotics. Finally I had a chance to visit the unit that would one day soon become my second home. When I first walked into the dialysis unit, I was so pleasantly greeted by the receptionist and the social worker took it from there, and gave me a tour of the facility. She answered my questions regarding my treatment, and my health insurance coverage. I then met the nurse manager of the unit, it was wonderful to meet her, because she gave me a run down of the unit; how long it's been in operation, the staff and what role they play in the comfort of each and every patient. I was introduced to some of the staff that were available and even some of the patients, who shared their stories about their first day, and how long they've been dialysis patients, of course a lot of them were veterans of many years of dialysis history. I was fascinated with some of them as to what they do to pass the time away; I noticed that some patients were watching the individual TV's provided for their enjoyment, some were listening to music on their walkman, some were talking to fellow neighbors next to them, and a lot of them were just simply catching zzzzzz. Or just chillin. I was then given my schedule and welcomed to my new family. My first day came, and I was called by name by who was to be my assigned nurse, this made me feel right at home and a little more at ease. After my weight, and vitals were taken, my needles were inserted and treatment began. My treatment was set for 2 ½ hours, and while having treatment, I didn't have to occupy my time to keep from getting bored, because one by one the nurse and technicians introduced themselves to me and welcome me to the unit. About an hour later, the dietitian came over and introduced herself, and ask me how was I feeling, she did expressed a concern for my mental state, if I was at all depressed because of the new change in my life. I assured her, that I wasn't. I began to tell her that I inherited the poly cystic kidney disease from my dad, so therefore I was quite condition to what was inevitable that happened to me. She continued on by discussing the renal diet with me, and how it will effect how well I do with kidney disease and dialysis treatment. The treatment time pass so fast that first day, with all the visiting from the staff and chatting with the patients that were in talking view of me. Actually my first day went very well, I didn't have one discomfort, but as the weeks went on, from time to time my treatments didn't run so very smoothly like they did that initial day. There are side effects from hemo dialysis treatment that I would experience from time to time, and I will share that experience with you later on in the book, but most importantly what causes these side effects with hemo dialysis treatment, such as: cramping of the body, and plummeting blood pressure.

My Family History of
Polycystic Kidney Disease

After enduring the trials and tribulations of my survival of poly cystic kidney disease with the blessing of the creation of dialysis, and after not learning much knowledge of the history of poly cystic kidney disease early on, I became curious to know, what exactly is poly cystic kidney disease, "wait a minute", before I keep spelling this disease out, I need to hip you readers to the abbreviation, PKD, which stands for poly (meaning many) cystic kidney disease for short. Now, on with the sharing of my family history. About a decade ago, I finally got around to researching to find out as much as I can about this PKD that has plagued my family in a very serious way. I traced it back as far as my Grandma Madea, who suddenly became ill and down south in those days, folks wouldn't see a doctor, unless their homemade remedies didn't solve the problem when it came to their health, however, she did eventually seek attention from a doctor, and after a series of testing, she was told that her kidneys were failing, but at that time, they didn't even tell her that she had PKD, I guess that is because, maybe they didn't have any knowledge of the exact name for what my Grandma was suffering from. She then took it upon herself to seek attention from a Voodoo doctor, who she thought may be able to help her get rid of whatever she had, but that proved unsuccessful. She was stricken with kidney failure in the late 1940's, and then finally in the early 1950's, she succumb to complications of the kidney failure, that resulted in the development of heart disease. Then finally in the early 1970's, my dad scheduled to have a hernia repaired after a physical, which while having the hernia repaired, it was discovered that my dad had the inherited kidney disease PKD, which by that time they knew what to call this kidney failure, and that is when my dad and his other siblings, knew exactly what their Mom had and had suffered from for all those years. I know that my dad inherited the disease from his Mom, but the twisted thing about all this, is that I don't know exactly who she inherited the disease from, which parent, her dad, the late Daniel White (aka Pa Dan), or her mom, the late Irene Picou (aka, Ma Lou), but there is a theory that it was on the White side of the family, because there are some relatives on my Granda Madea's dad side of the family, that have been stricken with PKD. I am still doing some ongoing research to trace beyond my Granda Madea, but still no success, but I will continue on my mission to go as far back as I possibly can, because there is still so much more unanswered questions as to when and where did this disease originated in our family history. Now, on with the story about my father's introduction to PKD and dialysis.

I will never forget the first time I heard the word **Dialysis**. It was one day when my mom and dad had returned from the city, from one of those mysterious trips they seem to be taking three times a week, (that us kids really didn't know what this trip was all about). All we knew was we weren't allowed to come along. And a visit to the city is very much a treat to us small southern town kids. Most of the time when we would frequent the city, it would be to go on a special shopping trip, or my parents had to see the dentist, other than that, there was no other reason to visit the city, because we lived about 50 miles outside the city. Our town was quite small and sort of in another world, so the city was like going to New York or Paris, or some exciting big city like that. Well anyway finally after many months of my sisters and I staying in the dark about their mysterious city trips, they finally decided to tell us about the coming events or shall I say changes that will take place real soon at home. Before they could tell us about the coming attractions, I immediately ask my dad, what is dialysis?, because I've heard them several times come back from their trip, saying the word *dialysis.*, I thought it was a very unique word. My dad promptly explains what dialysis is, and then he continues by telling us that he has been going to Charity Hospital in the city, for treatment and training at the same time. He explains to us that his kidneys have gone kaput, and he needs to have treatment from a machine, meaning the machine has to do the work his kidneys can no longer do. And this was going to happen real soon. He continued by telling us that a machine will soon be delivered and that we have some adjustments to make, meaning it could effect us as well as him, emotionally, mentally, and perhaps even financially. It was one Saturday morning, my sisters and I had just begun our summer vacation from school, and the delivery truck was at our door bright and early, right along with the record mobile, (that comes every other Saturday morning in our neighborhood selling the latest R & B tunes). You see the record mobile, as we kids call it, sold most of the R & B music, that other record stores didn't sell. Well anyway, this delivery truck had a lot of the neighbors and other folks on the street quite curious, as to what was being delivered, especially with a box of that enormous size, *Just nosey neighbors, you know, they are in everyone's neighborhood*. The machine could barely fit through the side door. It was set up immediately, because my dad was due to have a treatment that day. There really wasn't much time for small talk. My dad began to run the water hose through my bedroom window to the room where the machine was stationed. I don't know quite how much water had to be transferred to this machine, but it seem to be gallons and gallons of water drawn in that gigantic tank. I watched my dad go through this routine, first the drawing of the water, then the chemical check, he looked like a chemist measuring different vials and checking the contents of this mixture that he had to do every time he did the preparation that was necessary to do the treatment, in my opinion, all he really needed to play the part, is a white lab coat (LOL), well finally I know what the actual name for this machine is, the dialyzer, I don't need to refer to it as the machine through the continuation of this book. My dad would always explain things to me, because he knew I was always quite curious, so he tells me that the only reason he does the chemical check is to make sure the water is clear, and there is not a speck of blue (formaldehyde), running through the lines or tubing to be exact, that could be damaging and very harmful to him. After all the testing is done, Daddy had to have six slices of bread toasted and spread with butter. I really don't know why he craved this every time he was to do a treatment, but he wouldn't start a treatment without that toast bread and butter ritual. This went on for three years, even after I graduated from high school a year later. I remember there was a time when he was doing the prepping for his dialyzer, and I don't know exactly what caused the incident to happen, my mom was getting him ready to start treatment, you see she was trained to do the needle insertion, and she noticed when she connected the tubing to his arterial and venous line the solution was coming through the lines blue, and because of my mom's keen reaction she immediately clamped off the line. This could have seriously hurt my dad or even killed him. My mom realized my dad wasn't in his right mind, that the dialysis treatment was no longer functioning as well, this meant that the toxin wasn't being removed as well, and that it was staying in his blood and poisoning his system, causing issues with his thinking. Going through the motions, my going away to college, my dad became severely ill, the conclusion was he needed a kidney transplant as soon as possible, because the artificial kidney wasn't no longer doing its job. Through the grace of God his prayers were answered, and he received a cadaver (non-living donor kidney). It didn't function very long, because it wasn't one of those idea matches, that they have nowadays. When I look back on the circumstances of my dad's coping with dialysis, the dialyzer, the diet, and the procedure, It is so totally different from my first time dialysis. My dialysis life began almost two decades ago, I could almost remember it as though it happened yesterday. Seeing the dialyzer that was used for my treatment, is was very different from my dads big tank used at home. The first dialyzer I was on, it was no bigger than a large microwave oven, and it sat on a table right next to my recliner. I was being dialyzed at a outside unit. (that my dad wasn't fortunate to have during his saga of hemo dialysis treatment). This dialyzer wasn't very accurate, because most of the time I was never exactly at my dry weight after treatment, it was not very easy to calculate the right amount of fluid to take off. I was the majority of time very ill after treatment. Never feeling my best. Slowly the unit was beginning to get those upright computerized dialyzers. And after hounding my nephrologist about being changed to one of those new machines, finally one treatment I came in and I'm assigned to a new machine, I was so overwhelmed and flabbergasted, it was like a kid getting the best toy there is for Christmas. I look back and think the dialyzer went from a big tank to a microwave size dialyzer to now an upright computerized machine. It is great how much the dialysis world has advanced. Speaking of advancements in the dialysis world, I remembered when my dad was on hemo dialysis, he had issues with anemia, and to remedy that he had to have blood transfusions on a regular basis. I was more fortunate when it came to my blood, through the grace of god, EPO was created, and before I underwent a hemo dialysis treatment, I had to have a EPO shot once a week, until I started hemo dialysis. The advantage of having hemo, was the fact that I could get my EPO administered through my tubing during treatment, and those shots (that I truly despised) were no longer required. But now that I'm on peritoneal dialysis treatment, I had to go back to taking shots once a week. Looking back and how the renal world has advanced, many individuals like myself are living more longer, and productive lives than they were some forty years ago.

I also think back to the time when I first started dialysis, I praise God there were so many wonderful people that came into my life or should I say when I entered the dialysis world. I do miss my lunchtime round table discussion with what I called the "renal divas", each of us had very unique lives. Betty being the veteran of dialysis at our table, and plus she was the oldest in age, she was wise to the dialysis life, as well as everyday life in general. It was always quite a treat for me, being the youngest of the group and the rookie of the group as well. Betty would start the conversation off, by talking about how her treatment went, and then the other girls would chime in, and talk about their day, and even share home remedies for some of the problems that can arise with dialysis. Well I hadn't experienced any of those side effects, but as the weeks went on, I did finally experienced that drastic drop in blood pressure, that they had mentioned on occasion. It very much frightened me, I really don't know how you feel if you were dying, but I felt as though I was dying, because I had this weird feeling, and then I could hardly hear, and my vision was severely blurred, it gave me the feeling, like I was losing touch with reality. I began to panic, and was thinking what was happening to me, I'm I dying. I did yell out "I feel funny", and immediately a nurse charges over to me, and immediately reclined my chair, almost to the point that I was practically on the floor, this relieved some what, but I was also given a high dose of saline, I guess this was concentrated with an excessive amount of sodium (salt) hypertonic, I think they called it, if I'm not mistaken, however, I could taste it going through my veins. It wasn't very long before I was feeling better, to me it was remarkable how fast I came back to my old self. I must commend that nurse, because she was on the ball, didn't waste anytime bringing me relief. Now it is Friday, once again, and like clockwork me and the four renal divas met across the street at Pill Hill Café for lunch. This time one of the younger girls started off the conversation, with "Girl I was cramping my ass off" and at that point, I was wondering what she meant by she was cramping her ass off. I promptly interrupted her, and ask her why was she cramping, and of course, she and the rest of the group being experts at what to expect on dialysis, began to tell me that it is another side effect that you can get during and even right before the treatment is over. And I said is there a remedy for this, and why does this side effect have to happen? Well at that point, I was thinking this hemo dialysis ain't no joke, there is so much that I have to learn and experience, it's like going to medical school or something (LOL). Betty took it from there, and started explaining to me in detail why on occasions we can experience cramping. She told me that when you are in between dialysis sessions, you should watch your fluid intake in between treatments. We are told to very much limit our intake of fluids, because if we don't, we could experience a severe drop in blood pressure and plus those excruciating cramping pains. She also said that you can experience these cramps in any part of your body, she continued the conversation by stating that she tends to have them right in the back of the calf of her legs, and Donna, (another one of the girls in the group), remarked, I get them mostly in my toes and the balls of my foot. Maria, who happens to be of latin decent, said she gets them in her index and middle fingers. Then the rest of the girls joined in the conversation, it seems that these little lunch meeting were quite beneficial, and of course the girls felt a sense of relief talking about the haps on hemo. It seem to do them all the good just getting these stigmas off their chest. Joanne, was a little challenged, because she didn't really say much during our lunch sessions, but she would nod her head whenever someone talks about their mishaps, I guess that was her way of saying the same thing happens to her on occasion too. This really shade a little light on what my dad had to have been going through. I decided to put my little story into the mix, to try to fit in, I began to tell them about the stories of when my dad was on a home dialyzer, and when he would get these cramps in his leg, that would make his leg shoot straight up in the air. I told them how my two sisters and I would ride his leg to help him get rid of the cramps. This was like a treat for us kids, because we kids got a chance to ride what I called the ***human horse***. The girls got a real good kick out of this, they were practically fallen out there seats laughing. And that is when I felt like a part of the gang. And from that day on, I looked forward to those lunch meetings with the renal divas, just sharing stories and even sharing the occurrences of their personal lives. I truly felt gratified when I'm with these ladies, I learn so much from them to get a better grasp of this renal life. Now, the next Friday meeting seem to be geared towards the renal diet, that I soon discovered was very complex. I wanted to learn as much as I could about this diet, and any advice to help me in obtaining all the nutrients that I needed to continue maintaining my good health on dialysis. As time pass on, the routine Monday, Wednesday, and Friday treatment ritual continued, until about two years later, I was called for a transplant. Hallelujah!

My Transplant Experience

Now this was quite an exciting first time experience for me. Let me break down the scenarios that surround the day of the call. It was about 3:00 in the morning, and I had finally gotten to sleep, after a night of tossing and turning, and having serious insomnia, I finally got to sleep with the help of a benadryl pill. My mom was visiting my daughter and I, and she decided to take one of her benadryl pills to get some much needed sleep, also. Now, back to the call, the phone rangs, and I am like I said previously, in a daze, I answered the phone, and a very nice pleasant voice said these sweet words that was simply music to my hears, "Hello Ms. Jeff, this is the transplant coordinator at UCSF Transplant Center, Congratulations, you are the next candidate on our list for a cadaver kidney transplant. First, she was gracious enough to let me contain my composure, and to take in what was just relayed to me. She immediately, gave me instructions, to get to the hospital as soon as possible. Now, mind you, I was always prepared for this day, with my bag already packed, and any instructions on who was to take care of my toddler daughter, but that wasn't an issue, because my mom was, "thank God", visiting at the time. The only problem I had with getting ready, was that I was very drowsy from taking a benadryl hours before the call. My mom and I were dragging like zombies, she was trying to iron, and I don't know why she had to iron, she could have found something to wear that didn't need ironing, but anyway, that's my mom for you, what can I say. She was ironing in slow motion, and saying I don't know why I am going so slow with everything. And I said, could it be, because you are loaded off benadryl, (LOL) and she laughed sort of lazy like. I was having difficulty getting my own self ready, and then finally I struggled to get my toddler daughter ready, and of course she was acting so confused, saying mommy, "I'm sleepy, and I don't want to go". I truly didn't want to get into any drama with her, because to be honest with you, I didn't even have the strength, (LOL) even if I wanted to. I had to muscle up the energy to drag myself in the car, in which my boyfriend (at the time), who later became my husband, drove us to the hospital. I went straight to Admission, as I was instructed by the transplant coordinator. They were truly on the ball, my paperwork was there waiting for me at the front desk of Admission, I signed the necessary papers, and presented my insurance card, and driver's license, you know the drill. I was immediately instructed to go to the 6th floor, and as soon as I arrived, the nurse was waiting for my arrival, she escorted me to my room and told me to disrobe. I was amazed that I didn't have to wait very long after undressing, like you know, the usual long wait to be seem by the doctor, on a regular clinic visit. She began to take the usual vitals. It was great that I had just had a dialysis treatment early the day before, so my blood was pretty clean, and besides I hadn't eaten very much after treatment anyway. After all that was checked. I was having a lot of staff visitors during the night, such as: the neprologist (kidney specialist), surgeon, dietitian, and last but not least the anesthesiologist. The nurse came back and inserted an IV. Then about a few hours later, I was told it was time to go down to the OR. Boy, I had so much anxiety, my nerves were all in knots. I told the nurse, and she gave me IV meds to relax me, until I was wheeled into the OR. As soon as I got into the OR, I was shaved and scrubbed down very thoroughly. The RNs assisting with the surgery introduced themselves, and then the surgeon came in about 20 minutes later, and introduce himself. At the time they were playing some very mellow music in the background, it was very low, but I could hear it faintly. About 15 minutes later, the anesthesiologist entered the OR. He explained to me, the medication that he was to administer, and what it was for. After administering the general med, I was told to count from 100 backwards. I truly don't know how far backwards I had counted, before I was completely out, but when I finally was coming out of the anesthetic, I noticed I was in a totally different area of the hospital, which turned out to be the recovery room. I began to have discomfort from the incision, and was immediately told by the nurse, that I had a morphine pump, and I could administer my own medicine to relieve the pain. This was something that I had never had before, and it was a relief to not have to call for a nurse to give me something for pain, so I felt like I was in complete control. Really, to be honest with you, I didn't really have very much discomfort the next day after the surgery. I had a catherer, so I was urinating in the bag that was attached to my catherer. I hadn't urinated much in the last year, that when I saw how full the bag was, I guess that gave me an indication that my new transplanted kidney was doing its job, but when my neprologist came to see me, he did say that my labs indicated that my kidneys weren't working in full capacity. I was then told, that I needed some dialysis, about an hour to be exact. It was discovered that my AV Graft had clotted, and they decided to surgically place a subclavian (catherer) for temporary dialysis use. There wasn't much success in doing this surgery, it was a very blotched up procedure, which caused my neck to blow up like a huge tumor had taken over my neck. There was a sand sack like substance placed on my neck, and I was wheeled back to my room, and instructed to keep this sand sack placed on my neck, until the swelling subsides, and I was watched like a hawk by the nurse, for about six hours. When this was over, they decided to declot my Graft in my arm to be use for my dialysis. About three days later, I experienced my first rejection, and a biopsy was performed to find out how severe it was, I was given valium and benadryl before the procedure. After getting the biopsy results, I was diagnose with a minor rejection episode, but I was told that all the rejections are treated aggressively. I was given Tylenol and benadryl, before the actual anti-rejection drug was administered. I was given OKT3, (which is a very potent medication given by IV to prevent or reverse acute rejection episodes, this medication wipes out human white blood cells and stop them from attacking my new kidney). And about half hour after getting OKT3, I experienced side effects, which started with sweating, and then followed by uncontrollable shaking, in which they were aware that these side effects could occur, so they administered demoral, and it seem to work in a matter of minutes. I truly don't know what a drug addict actually goes through when it comes to withdrawals, but I really thought that I was going through some kind of withdrawals from this OKT3. Well after receiving this very powerful and strong anti-rejection drug, I returned to normal, meaning the rejection episode was over, and the fever subsided also, which indicated that there was no more sign of the rejection. A few days later, I started the training to learn to take the anti-rejection meds prescribed on my own, along with some white like tablet, that I had to place under my tongue for thrush. I had never heard of thrush before, so I immediately ask the nurse what was thrush, and she explained it to me by saying that it is a fungus infection that can develop in the mouth. I joked to the nurse, that I have to be very careful with so much with having this new kidney, even my mouth has to be protected, (LOL). I was also instructed that I needed to be aware of people that have herpes. There was so much to learn pre-discharge from the hospital. However, my stay was pretty lengthy, because I experienced yet another rejection, which the same protocol was taken, such as the biopsy to find out how severe the rejection was, and the results were a moderate rejection this time, but of course, all the rejections are treated aggressively like I mentioned previously, with Tylenol and benadryl to start, and of course that very powerful OKT3. When that was over, I had my labs redrawn, and the neph still had some concerns, about the kidney function, although I was urinating, where I wasn't doing very much of that, before the kidney transplant. During a visit from my daughter, mom and boyfriend, our daughter had to use the restroom, and of course a white hat was placed in the toilet, so that my urine output could be measured and tested, but this one time, when my daughter used the restroom, without my knowledge of her voiding in the white hat, the nurse removed the hat to be measured and tested, without my knowledge, and it came back with results that my kidneys were working at full capacity. I truly found this very strange, because it was only the day before that I still had to have some dialysis treatment, because of the lab results that were done the day before. So, when the nephrologist came to check on me, he wasn't too sold on these lab results either, so he ordered a redraw of my labs, and it came back with almost the same results that I had the day before. It was discovered that the urine that was tested from the hat, was truly from my daughter's output. All I could do was just laugh, because this was so funny to me, as well as my family and others in the room at the time. So, the next time when my daughter visited and had to use the restroom, I was sure to remind her to remove the white hat before she pee pee. Through all this, I was glad to have that morphine pump, whenever I had some pain or discomfort from the incision, but laughing as hard as I was, about this incidence with my daughter, I really needed that morphine pump more than ever., I was in so much pain from all this laughing, I even put a pillow over my incision, to kinda ease this pain a bit. About a week later, I wasn't to my surprise having any more pain or discomfort. It was getting close to a month, since my transplantation surgery, and finally my lab test were in normal range, so I didn't need anymore dialysis, Hallelujah!, I was preparing for discharge, which happen to occur on my birthday, isn't that something. Prior to being discharged, the nurse went over my meds, and made sure that I was instructed properly in following my medication schedule, along with what other meds I was taking previously before the transplant. She also made sure I was advised of when to visit for my two week checkup, and to always make sure several times a day, to utilize that large thick red band, that I was trained to use for regular exercising, during my hospital stay. I had been hospitalized for a month from the day of my kidney transplant surgery. I am one of those patients that truly don't like a wheelchair, but it was mandatory and hospital policy, that I be escorted out of the hospital in a wheelchair. As soon as my husband came around in the car to the emergency exit, where I was wheeled to, I hugged the nurse, (that I had gotten truly acquainted with during my lengthy stay at the hospital, and how kind she was to me, as well as other nurses at the hospital). I promptly got into the car, and was on my way home across the bay bridge to the east bay. It was exciting for me, to finally be out of the hospital, after so many weeks of just looking out the hospital window of the solarium (the name they called this room) right down the hall from my room. This room had a great city view of San Francisco and there was a little recreation in this room, with a big screen TV, VCR, and a couple of Nintendo games for the patients activity enjoyment, but I didn't miss it much, because I was so happy to be home. When I got out of the car, and into the sunlight, it seemed to give me a very funny feeling, I can't describe what this feeling truly felt like, but it felt as though I had to get reacquainted with being outside once again, I don't know, maybe if any of you readers have been in the hospital for a long time for one health issue or another, I mean more than three days stay, then you may know exactly what I am trying to express, (the feeling of being in the sunlight or daylight for that matter, after being cooped up for so many weeks in the hospital). At home, I was the comedian, because when I went on the toilet for the first time in a long time, to do the thing called <u>urinate</u>, Wow! I never thought I would ever say that word again, but I was actually <u>pissing</u>, (even this word too). (LOL). Well, anyway, I was urinating, and I was so excited about hearing this sound, that I hadn't heard in a very long time, well, even though I did hear it when my boyfriend would urinate (which always pissed up me off to the highest, because I could no longer piss, or for that matter, hear the sound of my own piss, but I am talking about hearing my own piss going in the toilet, for the first time, in a long time. I was so excited, that I didn't even close the door, when I used the toilet for the first time at home since being discharged from the hospital. I would say "Hey you guys do you hear it", and my mom and boyfriend replied, "Hear what?, I replied, me peeing, "ya hear it, "ya hear it", they thought I had lost my mind are something, but they really didn't understand how intrigued and excited I was hearing this very precious sound, but that wasn't the only crazy thing that was transpired that day, I even wouldn't flush the toilet immediately, because I wanted to just stare at it for a moment, before I flushed it down the toilet, I was saying to myself, "that's my piss", my piss in that toilet. This went on for weeks, until I got used to hearing and seeing the piss, but even though I didn't express it the same since the day I was discharged, every moment I piss, I was privately in mind, still excited to hear and see this beautiful liquid voiding all this toxin waste and excessive fluids from my body, and most importantly getting all the excessive minerals from my body, and balancing my phosphorus and calcium in my body. Not having to take those large phosphorus binders anymore. My diet became very friendly to me, I was eating all the potassium foods that I wanted, and the first thing I ate was, watermelon, and two baked potatoes, (with all the fixings, like crispy bacon, sour cream and steamed asparagus, (chopped in pieces), and of course shredded cheddar cheese), oh wow! Cheddar cheese, I could have cheddar cheese once again, as much as I can consume. Well, as the week went on, I had my first checkup appointment at the hospital, since I was going by car to the city, I didn't need the mask, like I was instructed to where, when I am out in public, because I didn't take any public transportation, and besides my mom, had that covered, because not only did she fumigate my apartment with Lysol, she sprayed the car with Lysol, so I didn't have to be concerned about germs of such. Oh, let me share with you what my mom would do to fumigate the apartment, she would take one of my large pots, like my huge Gumbo pot, and fill it half way with water, and then she would measure about a cup and a half of the liquid Lysol, and bring it to a boil, and then turn down the pot low to simmer. It would already be fumigating the kitchen, where it would be cooking, but then she would take it to the living room, and place the pot on a table, sort of in the middle of the room, but make sure that the pot has something under it, to not damage the furniture, or table, that the pot will be stationed on. I happen to have several wooden disk, that the pot would be foundation on, and pot of Lysol, would fumigate the whole apartment. Well, now lets get back to my visit to the hospital for my checkup. I remember during the time when I had the transplant, which was back in 1993, I was told to take my vitals everyday, twice a day, and keep these records, to bring to the appt. as a way for the doctor to see how well I was doing at home. My blood was drawn for an abundance of tests, such as electrolytes, (sodium, potassium, chloride, CO_2, and phosphorus), urea nitrogen (BUN), and of course, the creatinine. There was other test being drawn such as CBC (complete blood count) - you know the hematocrit to monitor anemia, hemoglobin - to monitor blood oxygen level, platelets - to monitor bleeding tendencies and WBC (white blood count) - infection/rejection. Glucose (sugar) - to monitor pancreas function, because I was told earlier on, that anti-rejection meds could cause steriod induced diabetes, so the immunosuppressive blood levels need to be monitored very closely for the levels of immunosuppressive drugs in my body, and of course PT (prothrombin time) - to monitor blood clotting in my body. The amylase also helps in monitoring the pancreas function. I was very familiar with these test, once I became a transplant recipient, because I previously was employed as a chemistry clerk, and a great deal of these test, I was familiar with, working in a hospital chemistry lab, I even knew a great deal of the abbreviation for some of the minerals, that I really didn't dream possible would become important to me in regards to my health, Go Figure! These are life's challenges that I never thought I would have to face, but I am so grateful to God, that I worked in that capacity, because believe me, it was very beneficial to me, to better understand the scenarios that I faced with my transplant with lab values, and how important they were to my transplant. That was truly a blessing for me, to have that knowledge of laboratory terms. If I knew medical terminology, then I know I would be set, right!. I know there are more test that are drawn, but if I continue to list more test, this book will become boring with a lengthy lab test listing. The one thing that was very important, that the nurse instructed me to do, was when I had my clinic appointments, I was not to take my cyclosporine before my blood draw, she told me to remember to bring it with me, and take it after my blood was drawn. There was more protocol to keep in mind, when it came to my medication regiment, I was told to always have a least one week's supply of medication on hand. However there was a group of us patients scheduled each time that I would have my checkup to be examined and have blood drawn. The routine started with the lab draw, 30 minutes before the actual clinic appointment, I then checked in with the clinic clerk (personal), she handed me a urine container for my urinalysis testing. This was also wonderful to me, to be given a cup to void in, and I didn't have to no longer strain to get any piss out, I didn't even have to let the water run in the sink, to get the urge to piss. (lol). Of course my blood pressure, weight and temperature was checked. Later a physical exam was done by the doctor. The doctor then reviewed all my medication (checking the indication and dosage). After I had gone through all this protocol, the doctor provided me with a slip of paper, which indicated the next clinic date, I was then instructed to give this paper to the front desk clerk, so she could record and schedule this next appt. date. My nephrologist informed me that he would look over the lab results after clinic and call me that afternoon or the next morning with my results. During the first few months, I had many frequent follow up appointments, this didn't taper off until a few months after the transplantation. I am truly not sure how much this has all changed in the many years after my transplantation, but this is the protocol that I was instructed to follow, but we know that things can change in the medical industry in a decade and seven years, since my transplant. Although, I only embraced the pleasure and blessing of having this cadaver kidney, for four months, it was just great having any kind of a break from dialysis treatment, whether it be a few years to a few months. Now as I was home enjoying my new blessing (the cadaver kidney), about the fourth month of having this transplant, I had symptoms of a possible rejection, first my temperature began to rise, and I took Tylenol to bring it down, but it spiked right back up in a matter of a few hours. I also began to have a very weird symptom, my feet seem to turn inside out sort of, I knew something was wrong, so I immediately called the transplant center, and told them what was happening with me, and I was instructed to immediately go to the ER dept, at the hospital that I had the transplant as soon as possible, it was obvious that I couldn't drive myself, so one of my good friend, Phil, (and it so happen to be the middle of the night). I promptly phoned him in a panic, and he didn't hesitate to come to my rescue. After I arrived, they knew exactly what to do. My vitals were taken, such as my temperature, and blood pressure. The labs were taken, and when the results came back, it was an indication that I could possibly have a rejection going on, so a biopsy was done. This result came back immediately, and I was told that I was having a very severe rejection (meaning major). It was during the Christmas holiday season, so a surgeon had to be summoned, and because the hospital rooms were all booked up, I was allowed to stay in the ER overnight, until the on-call surgeon arrived, which took about two and half hours. Because I was to have emergency surgery, I was NOP (not allowed to eat anything before the surgery). Finally, the surgeon arrives, and I am promptly prepped for surgery. After the surgery was over, I think it took several hours for the removal of the cadaver kidney, my native kidneys remained. You know the scenario, I was in the recovery, and then admitted to a room. I guess I was in and out, all through the night. The very next day when I was

more alert, the nephrologist scheduled a test to check my native kidneys,
I guess to see what was going on with the cyst on my kidneys, but this
was a very devastating time for me. After this procedure was done, I was
wheeled into the waiting area of this department, and as I was waiting for
the orderly to take me back to my room, I was starting to experience
breathing difficulty, it was to the point, that I could hardly breathe. I
noticed there were other medical staff sitting around, and I tried to get
their attention, that I had breathing difficulty, but it wasn't easy for me
to yell, or even speak for that matter. I tried waving my arms at them, but
they weren't paying no attention to me, so I got furious, and saw a waste
basket right next to my wheelchair, so I muscled up some strength to pick
that waste basket up, and throw it at the reception desk window, and that
is when I got their attention, that I was in distress. They abruptly looked
over at me, and I guess being medical professionals themselves, knew
right then and there, that I was having breathing difficulties. From there,
they took me to a room, and because I already had an IV in place, I was
immediately administered some kind of sedative. After about two weeks,
I finally awakened, and the nurse that was at the time changing my IV
fluid bottle, saw that I had awakened, and she said "welcome back", and
I looked at her very confused, and said "welcome back from where?", and
she continued by explaining to me, what occurred during these two
weeks, that I truly don't have any memory of, you have been mostly
sleeping for over two weeks in a comatose state, meaning I was in and out
of consciousness, during that time. She did say, that since you have
awakened, they may stop your IV fluid, and start you on a liquid diet,
and then a full course diet. What I do remember was, not too long ago, I
was eating a very normal diet, and now I am told that I am back on a
strict renal diet, that is when I slowly remembered what lead me to be
admitted to ICU. And remembering that I lost the kidney transplant, I
began to remember, what transpired, right before this ICU admission. I
started singing like a canary, when it all came back to me, I shared the
story with nurses, x-ray tech, my roommate, and even housekeeping. I
even shared it with a nurse, who claimed to be Oprah Winfrey's aunt. She
told me this, one day, when I was watching Oprah's talk show. Well, after
talking all day, non-stop about this incidence, that happened after a CT
Scan, the next morning, I couldn't hear, and for a whole day, I couldn't
hear, the nephrologist, examined me, and I was told that this could be a
side effect from the medication, that I was on, while in ICU. What
follows next, a few days later, I couldn't speak, I would open my mouth,

and not a sound would come out, now I am truly freaking out more, I press the nurse call button, but when she responded, I couldn't speak, and I tried so very hard to bring this to her attention, until finally I took a pen, that I had been doing a word search game, and hit the call button real hard, and she responded, what is that noise, Ms. Jeff, is anything wrong, not getting a response from me, she rushed over to my room, and because I couldn't speak, I began to write, that I lost my voice somehow. She immediately called for doctor. It took about an hour, before he came to my room. I guess the nurse had to page him. He examined me once again, and came to the same conclusion, about the lost of hearing issue, a possible side effect of the medication used. He left and came back, but he had an audience with him, some interns, I guess they were there to observe me. He began to ask me certain questions, like do you know where you are, and who is the President of the United States, I answered those questions promptly, but when he ask me what was the date, I didn't answer right away, because my mom was in the back of the doctor, pointing (on the sly) at the calendar on the wall, as though this was about me getting the right answer, to receive a passing grade or something, but I did answer it right, by watching my mom point at the calendar. They were asking these questions, to find out if I suffered any brain damage from this comatose state, that I had been in for almost two weeks. He then ordered a MRI procedure, to see indeed, if I had suffered any brain damage, or even a stroke during this time. Because of what I previously experienced with having a CT Scan, after the MRI testing was completed, I was wheeled right on the outside of the MRI room, and placed there to wait for an orderly to take me back to my room, ten minutes had passed, and it felt like I was in that same situation with the CT Scan, which left me with difficulty trying to breathe remember!, well, finally the orderly arrived, and took me back to the room, only to find out that my mom felt like it was taking too long for me to be taken back to my room. She asked the nurse about my whereabouts, and she did express that she knew what happened when I had the CT Scan procedure, and she didn't want this to happen again, she began to pressure the nurse to have an orderly come to get me as soon as possible. I was flattered, that my mom is the reason why I didn't have to wait very long, before an orderly was there to take me back to my room. Actually she came for a visit, about ten minutes after I left for this MRI testing, and I guess she thought it was way too long to still be down at the MRI room going through that procedure. At this time, my mom only knew about my hearing issues, and she was surprised to witness that I couldn't utter a word, not one word. She looked at me with a very weird look, when she ask me how was I feeling, and I couldn't tell her, I just wrote on my steno tablet, "I feel O.K., but I have lost my voice", and she promptly said in a very angry term "what! You can't talk", then she followed by saying " not at all", and I nodded no. When the neprologist began to make his rounds, he entered the room, and immediately realized that I still couldn't speak, but my hearing had returned. He replied, "your voice hasn't been restored", and my mom abruptly ask the nephrologist what he thinks caused this?, and of course, he stated the very same thing he told me, was he believed it was a side effect from all the meds I was on during my comatose state. The whole day, I couldn't speak, and after a good nights sleep. I woke up that morning, I yarned with noise, so I knew right then and there, that my voice had returned. One day without speaking does effect a person in a very serious way, especially if they are use to talking a lot, like myself, I was anxious to try my restored voice out on someone, so I pressed the nurse call button, and she answered, it brought so much joy to me, to be able to respond, nothing, I was just trying out my vocal chords, and she of course, not being the nurse that was on duty, when I had this not being able to speak episode, thought it was very strange what I had just said to her on the speaker box. She came over, I guess just because I responded with nothing, and etc, etc., she came to the room only to find me, saying I can speak, and she responds yeah! And!, well let me just clarify, Just a day ago, I couldn't utter a single word, not even a sound of such, and she said I wasn't aware of this. Well, because of all this, I didn't want to eat, but when my voice was restored, I told the nurse, that I was starving, and because I missed breakfast, she had a snack tray ordered. I noticed that my AV Graft was declotted, and I was once again back to three days a week hemo treatments, but I wasn't well enough to be discharged. I got a call from some dear friends, who was glad to find that I was doing alright, but they didn't hesitate to ask, if I had an out of body experience, and I went what! Why would you ask that, so they said my boyfriend, mentioned to them, that I was in a comatose state for almost two weeks, but I assured them, that I don't remember any out of body experience. Now, I have been hospitalized for three weeks at this time, and Christmas was quickly approaching. I hated being in the hospital for Christmas, they had what they call a skeleton crew, (staff that I had never seen before), and they weren't very kind to me, and maybe it was because they had to work on Christmas., I guess. However, my boyfriend visited, and brought

Christmas gifts for me, and it made the day, a little more enjoyable and satisfying. One of the gifts, was a cassette player, and I was happy about that. After that, my mom and daughter called and wish me Merry Christmas, this made me so very sad. Finally, I was ready to be discharged, but this time I wasn't very excited about going home, because I didn't have the cadaver kidney no longer. Returning to the dialysis unit for treatment, I was in a very bad mood, it took a few weeks, before I accepted the fact that it was back to dialysis business as usual.

Returning to Hemodialysis

When I returned to the dialysis unit, I discovered that one of the Renal Divas from our roundtable discussion group wasn't with us, and I ask Betty, where was Donna, and I was told that she went on a trip to Texas, for a family union. About a month passed, and I became very concerned about Donna, and finally a few days later she returned, but without both of her legs. I was happy to see her, but not to see her in that condition. She told me her legs were amputated, because of a sore, that wouldn't heal properly, and I truly felt sorry for her. She did admit that it was her fault, because she wasn't taking good care of herself, during this trip, but one thing about Donna, that I admired, was she hadn't lost her sense of humor. She would say, I guess I'll be sitting down a lot, however, I am considering getting artificial legs. Well that is wonderful prospect, I replied. Now, two years has passed since the transplant, and my boyfriend and I were considering moving away from the city, because during the time of my kidney transplant, my daughter sort of rebelled, she was beginning to not do well in school, especially when I decided to let her go back to Louisiana with mom, to live for awhile. We moved to a suburb right outside the city, and of course, I had a new adjustment to make, especially at a entirely different unit. After settling into our new home, I soon miss my previous neprologist, because I noticed things were done so much different from the unit that I went to in the city. I wasn't very happy with this move, when it came to this new dialysis unit, which was way smaller than the unit in the city, it had only about ten stations, but the one thing that was great about it, is everyone practically new everyone there. Even though I lost the transplanted kidney, I was still having issues with swelling, after returning to hem dialysis. Now, after becoming a patient at the new unit, my edema issues became a very serious problem, that my new neprologist thought it would be less taxing on my body, if I had two Grafts in usage, I could rotate them every other day, but this wasn't the solution, I was still having major problems with edema, so much, that I had this very hideous looking appearance. Even with all this edema going on, I had to have repairs to my

Graft, having angioplasties, because of artery blockage, having stents and balloons put in place.

Finally, I had, had my third graft, and I was told that I could no longer have grafts placed in the upper part of my body, so I resulted to a fourth graft, (a leg graft), placed on the left thigh. This leg graft, proved to be as taxing as having grafts in the upper part of my body, especially when it burst twice on me, it was a very devastating time for me, having numerous surgical procedures to repair this graft, finally after two years, this final graft failed, (more of this graft experience is in my first published book - "My Renal Life (I know it, I live it). Well, finally after four failed AV grafts, I had to transition to peritoneal dialysis treatment.

My Transition from Hemodialysis to Peritoneal Dialysis

Now, before I continue sharing this particular experience, let's get acquainted with the abbreviation for peritoneal dialysis (PD). Now, on with the story, like I mentioned in the previous chapter - my return to hemo dialysis, after the lost of the transplanted kidney, remember! Well, this transition didn't go as smoothly as it could have. Due to the trauma that I suffered from my leg graft, I could no longer have any access for hemo dialysis. While still having hemo dialysis treatments, I was also being trained by the PD nurse, Tyra LaChappelle, to transition to PD in a matter of weeks, but due to a complication with the surgery of my last graft, (the leg graft), it wouldn't heal properly, I had to constantly have surgery to relieve the problem that I was having with the leg surgery, where the Jackson Pratt, (a device tubing, that was placed to drain the inflammation (pus) that would collect in my leg), it wasn't doing its job, and I had to have several emergency surgeries to drain the inflammation from my leg. It was collecting in my leg, and not in the device that was placed in my leg for that purpose. Finally, after a month, the surgeon found a way to drain my leg permanently, and guess where they had to go, to solve this, the surgeon had to go in my foot, (my big toe to be exact) to finally remedy this surgical problem. But even though this problem was remedied, I had to start my first PD treatment in the hospital, and I soon discovered that the nurses were very rusty with this treatment. I always give prop to my PD nurse, Tyra, for her very precise training and of course all the notes that I took during this training. Seeing that the nurse was rusty with this, I did the manual exchanges by myself, first, when they warmed the PD solution, it was way too hot, when I felt it, and they had to start all over again, warming it. This time it was O.K., to go ahead with the exchange. Because I didn't have any dwelled solution to drain, all I did was fill my peritoneum with 2000, with a 2.5 dextrose strength. And after a four hour dwell, the nurse warmed the ultra bag perfectly, and I was able to drain, fill and then dwell with much success, no pain or discomfort whatsoever. I was so proud of myself with my initial treatment. During this time, I was reporting back to my PD nurse, Tyra, about how I was coping with PD, and making sure I was doing all preparation and steps properly, and she assured me, that I was coming along fine, she did say that she has every confident, that I could handle this very well. This truly gave me, much confidence, that I could do very fine with, PD. I did two days of PD, and then I was finally discharged. I continued that afternoon, with my next PD treatment, and everything went well. About a month and a half of this, it became a little too tedious for me, I felt like I was ready for the training of the night time cycler PD treatment. This training went very well, and I will share with you the way this treatment is done, first there is a machine required for this treatment, and I do five exchanges a night, which is a total of ten hours straight.

Preparations and Instructions
Of
Manual Exchanges of Peritoneal Dialysis Treatment

Step by Step Instructions:

Ultra Bag Exchange Procedure:
1. Secure the Area, used to do the PD exchange
2. Make sure the surface is clean, that you will be using
3. Collect supplies, check ultra-bag for: concentration, leaks, amount, date - CLAD
4. Warmed ultra bag, two clamps, mini-caps, and mask
5. Have transfer set easily accessible
6. Mask on
7. Wash hands thoroughly with antibacterial soap, don't touch anything with your hands after they are washed, use a paper towel to place your hands on the faucet and doorknobs
8. Clamp two (2) lines: fill line and drain line
9. Break - 2 areas of the transfer set - dialysate and Y tubing segment
10. Connect sterile transfer set and sterile Y tubing segment, then the mask can be removed
11. Flush: Unclamp both line clamps count to 2 slowly then clamp both lines
12. Drain: Open transfer set, open drain line clamp, until there is no more fluid movement, clamp drain line
13. Fill: Open fill line clamp, until prescribed amount of dialysate has flowed from bag to the patient
14. Close fill line clamp, and transfer set
15. Mask on

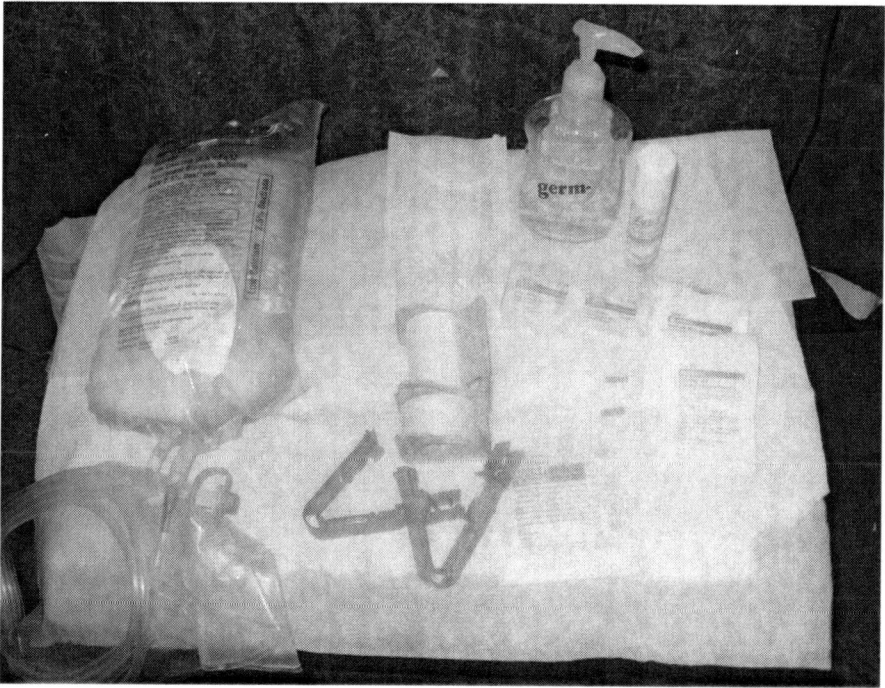

16. Wash hands, use a hand sanitizer
17. Open one of the mini cap, be sure it is in close reach
18. Disconnect - Sterile Y tubing segment from the transfer set, just drop the Y tubing segment. Place mini cap on transfer set
19. Check drain bag, solution should be clear
20. Discard used equipment properly

Being trained for the nightly cycler treatment, is totally different. It took a couple of weeks to be trained and most importantly be confident enough to finally do the treatment at home on my own. Although I have been doing the cycler for almost ten years now, I could remember my initial start at home. First, I made up a chart of the step by step, cycler treatment directions, and of course, I forgot to mention that I did the very same thing, when I started my manual exchanges at home (I created a poster with step by step directions). Starting the cycler, I was more of a nervous wreck, than when I first started the manual exchanges. I purchased a table, that I felt was very appropriate for my cycler machine. First, of course, the bags were a little too heavy for me to pick up, so my husband places the two bags on the cycler, (they are 6000L bags), and the heater bag is a 2.5 dextrose strength, while the second bag, which is placed on the convenient slide table, that is attached to the main table, (I told you this was the perfect table for my cycler), which is a 1.5 dextrose strength. When the heater bag is warm, about ten to fifteen minutes, I continued with the prepping of the cycler. The display panel, which lights up in green, displays - PRESS GO TO START - then it will display in green also, LOAD THE SET, (Transfer Set), make sure all the clamps are close, (there is five clamps, red, blue, three white clamps, make sure the drain bag or drain line is connected to the drain line tubing. Press go again and it will display SELF TESTING, and after that steps is completed, it will display CONNECT BAGS, connect the bags with the device provided to connect the bags safely. After this step is completed, open three of the clamps, the red clamp (the heater), second bag clamp, and the patient line, then press the go button again, and it will display - PRIMMING, and this goes for about ten minutes, and when that is completed, it will alarm, and it will display - CONNECT PATIENT, and that is the complete protocol to setting up the machine. A very simple and painless procedure. Although this is a very simple and easy way to dialyze, there are times that a patient could experience a few minor glitches, and believe me I have had my share during these ten years that I have been doing PD for treatment. I will share a few of these mishaps that I have had. When I first started on the cycler, I was having very bad excruciating pain, whenever I would fill, it was soon apparent, that when I would do my initial drain, that it would drain me dry, and when I would fill, my tubing would dangle inside me, which will cause this pain. I brought this to the attention of my PD nurse, and she told me to bring my cycler in, so she could change it to something called TIDAL, which it will leave a small overflow, so that when I fill, the tubing wouldn't dangle, as much, while I am in my fill mode of the exchange, well not so much, that it could continue to give me pain. It has been set this way ever since, and I haven't had any discomfort for the pass ten years of PD, but don't get me wrong, I do have my share of problems with my cycler, such as alarms for low patient flow. I remember when I first started the cycler, which almost two years ago, I still this day, share my humble beginning with other fellow dialysis patients, (who could be considering PD as their form of dialysis, or those like me, who maybe considering a transition from hemo to PD), whatever the case, I don't mind sharing my humble beginning with others. My humble beginning after a few months of manual PD exchanges, I grew tired of the every four hour deal, so I decided it was time to consider the night time cycler for continued PD treatment. Starting the cycler, I was a nervous wreck, when it was time to this, on my own at home. I first made up a chart, (just like I did with the manual exchange), I would refer to this list, for awhile, until I had became familiar and comfortable with the prepping of the cycler. Well, anyway, my dilemma came, when I had to figure out, where I was going to sleep, during the cycler treatment. I decided not to sleep in the bed, the first night, I slept in my recliner, that I was sitting in, when I would do my manual exchanges, but that didn't last, but a couple of nights, because it wasn't a very comfortable way to sleep, and besides I had alarms all night long, and it was mainly - check the patient line, which I wasn't positioned properly, because the cycler kept detecting this. I would like turn sideways, and this seem to solve the problem, but it wasn't very comfortable for me, so I didn't get any sleep that first night. I decided after two nights, of nothing but alarm after alarm, that I would sleep in my bed. Oh, I forgot to tell you about my husband having to put the bags on the cycler for me, because they proved to heavy for me to be lifting. My total volume for treatment was 11,000ML, when I first started, but that changed through the years, from time to time, and I will tell you later on, why on occasion, the prescription would change.

Here is a breakdown of my individualized prescription for the PD cycler machine: *Note: every PD patients prescription is different, it is based on their weight, nature of the development of chronic kidney disease, other health issues, and remaining kidney function.*

Total Volume - 11,000ML
Therapy Time - 10 (ten) Hours
Fill Volume - 2000ML
Total UF - 400ML
Last Fill - 1000ML

My bags were a 6000ML - equivalent to 12000ML - which it took two bags to get my total prescription of 11,000ML
Dextrose Strength that I use normally - 2.5 and a 1.5
1.5 - the weakest strength
2.5 - standard strength
4.25 - the strongest strength - and it is recommended, only to use this strength on occasion, (if the blood pressure is quite elevated) - because too much usage of 4.25 can damage the pancreas
Cycles - 5 total, which mean these steps: drain, fill, and dwell, are done five times during the night - which totals the 10 hour therapy
Last Fill - 1000ML - (Note: some people are fortunate, not to have a last fill)
Dwell Time - 1 hour 33 minutes, but this does change from time to time, especially, if a patient is experiencing alarms during the night

Also, I have to do a daytime manual exchange as a part of my prescription, now, there some patient that are fortunate enough to not have to do a manual exchange. I don't urinate much, since starting PD, so that determines whether I need to do a manual exchange. There are so many factors that determine how the patients PD prescription is setup.

Now, back to the initial first month of night time cycler treatment. Setting up the cycler on a table of some sort, was a task for me, I tested various tables, until I purchased this one table from IKEA, it was the idea table for my cycler. I feel in my opinion, if you have a table that is level to your bed, (which is level to your body), it works so much better with the flow of the solution from your body, (draining, as well as filling). Oh, now getting back to that perfect table (in my opinion), for my cycler. The table also has a side table, that folds to the side, when not in use, I use this side table to place the second bag on. I also have a drawer, right below the table, and right below that, is a metal type basket, that I store needed mini caps, alcohol preps, betadine, syringes, surclens (a solution used to clean the PD catherer and surrounding area), mask and gloves (to use when necessary). There is also a third metal drawer, that slides out, and I store my bottles of medicine, Icy Hot, ace bandages, vapor rub, and anti-itching lotion. Now, back to the treatment. There was this one time, when I didn't do a manual exchange, because I was out and about, passed the schedule time for my manual exchange, so I opted not to do the exchange, and go straight to my nightly cycler treatment, but during the initial drain, my drainage amount was very low, because the cycler, kept alarming, looking for at least 1000ML as an output, but I only drained about 700ML, because apparently, when I dwelled passed the time of my midday manual exchange, while I was dwelling, my body absorbed a great deal of the solution, that I was dwelling, which was 1000, because that was my set last fill. I hope you can understand what I am talking about. Because of the low initial drain, the cycler, kept alarming, and after two times, I decided to finally call the Baxter helpline to assist me, with a solution to this problem, they ask me what mode of the exchange I was in, and I told them I have never gotten out of the initial drain mode, so they continued by asking what my initial drain setup was, and I told them, so they immediately came to the conclusion, that I must have absorbed a great deal of my last fill, during the dwell time. I was then told to *BYPASS*, and they gave me the instructions step by step on how to do this. After that, the rest of the night went very well, but every time, I was naughty, and stayed out pass my schedule dwell time, I knew that my schedule didn't allow me to do a manual exchange, so I went on with the cycler treatment, but this time, I was aware of why I got that slow patient flow alarm, and I knew exactly what to do, *BYPASS*. The important fact about *BYPASS*, is that it is not always safe to do, so be very sure it is safe to *BYPASS*, just check with the *BAXTER* helpline, and they will tell you, if it is safe for you to *BYPASS*. When I would get a *CHECK DRAIN LINE*, I would go through the check line steps - and check for such things as: kinks in the tubing or bag port, closed clamps, fibrin blockage, and when I would find fibrin in the drain bag, or in the drain line, (you can see fibrin floating through the tubing - it looks something like cotton floating in the tube) - I would put heparin in the heater bag - step by step - first I would put my mask on and this time a pair of gloves, and get the vial of heparin and syringe ready, I would take a betadine pad, and wrap it around the heater bag port, and hold it there for about fifteen minutes, and then I would also do the same for the top of the heparin bottle, and then I would take the syringe and insert the amount of heparin, needed for my particular heparin prescription, and then I would insert it into the port of the heater bag, and wait five minutes for it to circulate through the bag, then press go to continue the therapy. Oh, also remember, to stop the therapy, when you have to administer heparin, so that you will not lose any of your therapy time. On and on, with the night time cycler exchange. Now, I did have some problems when it came to the draining of the PD solution. When I first started I was using the drain line, but that proved a problem with the plumbing in my home. There was the one time in the beginning, when I used the drain line, and I had some very severe flooding, I was putting the drain line in the toilet, and I didn't know at the time, that when this drain solution goes into the toilet, and when it gets airborne, it turns into a jell like substance, which clogged my pipes, and it back up, and water was leaking to the downstairs room. I decided right after that incidence, to only use drain bags, because the only reason, this flooding happened, is because, if a patient uses a drain line, they have to flush the toilet through the night, so that the solution can't sit and get airborne, and this flooding mishap can be avoided. My husband decided that when he is discarding my drain bag, and any remaining solution that wasn't used, that he needed to keep our pipes clear, and he has been flushing the pipes with something called *Rid X*, and it has worked ever since, in keeping our pipes clear, no more flooding or plumbing problems, so keep in mind, about all this, when it comes to your pipes, my home has very old pipes, so if any of you readers out there, decide on PD as your choice of dialysis, keep this in mind. Finally, after five years of PD treatment, I developed peritonitis, (an infection that can develop from PD - somehow germs were introduced into the peritoneum) - it could be from an infection around the PD catherer, where a patient could have trauma, from some pulling of the catherer site, or germs could have gotten through, from the connecting or disconnecting of the mini-cap, go figure!, I just don't know when those little rascals could have gotten in, there is such a small window, when it comes to the connecting and disconnecting of the mini-cap, you ready have to pay serious close attention, when you come to this step in the PD therapy process, there could be so many scenarios as to how a infection can develop. Well, I got my first episode of peritonitis, during a trip, and I do believe, that I got it from a hotel stay. (*Keep in mind, and I can't stress this enough, that there is a very short window for connecting and disconnecting from the bags, whether it be manual exchange or cycler exchange. Just be safe, sanitary, and most importantly quick about this step of the pd process).* Now, back to my first episode of peritonitis, I returned home, and I did a manual exchange, and I noticed the bag was a little cloudy, and of course, my blood pressure was plummeting, which followed by shaking, and then I took my temperature, and yes, I was running a fever. I went to the unit, to be administered some antibiotics, but about an hour after getting their standard antibiotic, I broke out in a rash, and it was soon apparent that I had a allergic reaction to this medication. I immediately went to ER, and of course, they went through the protocol, that they follow, such as take some fluid from my peritoneum, and test the white blood count (WBC). I already knew I had the infection, but that is the protocol, that the ER has to follow. I did however, learned something from this first experience, is that if you have to go to ER, as I did, because you maybe allergic to the standard antibiotic used at the unit, it would be wise if you would take your last manual exchange to the ER, to be tested, because I noticed the ER nurse was very careless with the procedure of taking the fluid from me to be tested, but of course, I already knew I had peritonitis, so I wasn't as concerned at that time, about the safeness of doing this procedure, but it was something to be cautious about in the future, just in case, if I was to develop another infection, I would bring the last exchange in for testing, because this would speed up the process of being admitted and the nurse can start administering the antibiotics as soon as possible. Now, back to my stay in the hospital, because of my very low blood pressure, I was admitted to ICU, so they could monitor my blood pressure much more closely and frequently. First, while I was in ER, I was given albumin intravenously (IV), and moments later, I started feeling real funny, first, my vision suddenly became blurred, and then I could faintly hear, and that is when the nurse quickly took my blood pressure, and that was an indication that my blood pressure had dropped drastically low. They put me in ICU, and began administering an antibotic by IV, which the following day, I discovered that my throat felt like it was closed off, Wow! I am aware of some of my allergies to some antibiotics, such as penicillin, amphicillin, and vancoymcin (discovered from getting this med at the dialysis unit). This new antibiotic, was a very new allergic reaction. My neprologist immediately stopped this antibiotic, started me on a new antibiotic, and that seem to work, I wasn't showing any signs of any allergic reaction to this particular medicine, I was also administered two more antibiotics. I had a four day stay (two days in IUC, and two more days in a private room). Continuing to have intravenous antibiotics and blood draws several times of day. During this hospital stay, I didn't have much of an appetite, and besides the hospital food I didn't particular like, so that made it even more difficult for me to gain an appetite. I struggled to just eat anything on my plate to get some much needed nutrients. However, I don't think it was so much that I didn't have an appetite, because when my daughter came to visit and spend the night, she brought some chicken from home, and as soon as I smelled the aroma from this chicken, my appetite came back full force, I just snuck a chicken breast, which that was the healthiest piece to eat for my strict renal diet, you know, to watch the cholesterol intake, do you know after I ate that chicken, later on during the night, when they took my blood pressure, the nurse was amazed, at how my blood pressure had risen, because she was concerned about me earlier on, saying you need to eat something, because your blood pressure is way too low, but it was obvious, that restriction of sodium intake from my diet, was the problem, because it was evident, that I needed some salt, to help bring my blood pressure up, but you know that when you are in the hospital, and you are a dialysis patient, it is mandatory to restrict the sodium in the renal diet. I was finally being discharged, but with instructions to continue taking two of the antibiotics at home. Now mind you, my blood pressure wasn't exactly in normal range, but it had elevated enough for me to be discharged. Taking the antibiotic at home, proved to me, that it is what was causing me to have such a funny appetite, and I was also still experiencing low blood pressure. This went on for another two weeks of antibiotics, and after finishing all the antibiotics, I had a culture down at the unit, and the results came back with a very low WBC. About a few days later, I noticed my appetite was getting better and better, and of course, my blood pressure soon began to rise, so I stopped the 1.5 solutions, and was back to the normal PD prescription of 2.5 bags. Now, I am the kind of dialysis patients, that want to learn from my issues with certain meds, so I documented all that I had endured during my two weeks at home, antibiotic ritual. Like they say, you learn from your experience or mistakes, (if that is the case). Well, on with the usual PD treatment regiment. I won't share my PD experience from a day by day perspective, but some of what I experienced, could happen to you. About a year, after starting PD treatment, I started having pain on my left side, and because I was warned by my PD nurse, Tyra, to beware of peritonitis, I thought this symptom indicated that I may have developed an infection, however, I did check my bag for cloudiness, but that wasn't apparent, I continued by checking my temperature, and I was running a slight fever, so I decided right then, to go to ER, since it was the late evening. Since I was experiencing excruciating pain, and I told the ER nurse, that I may have peritonitis, be advised, that if you go to ER and tell ER, that you are a PD patient, and you may have symptoms of peritonitis, it takes priority in ER, they take you right in, because I was told early on, that it is important to get medical attention for peritonitis as soon as possible. Well, after being promptly taken to a room, I was still having those excruciating pains in my left side, they did the necessary protocol to test my PD fluid, and while waiting for the results, I became nauseated, and ask for a barf basin, and yes I did throw up, but it wasn't food, it was blood clots, and that is when the nurse said "I think I know exactly what is going on with your body. She immediately reported this to the attending ER physician, and he ordered a procedure that could scope my stomach. I was administered an IV med, to put me to sleep, this was all happening in the ER room, and the nurse, was surprised that the sleeping med didn't take effect right away, she kept saying remarks like "she's still not getting sleeply! so the nurse administered a little more, continued saying "I never seen this medication work so slow any other patient before. Finally, I fell into a deep sleep, I don't know how long it took, but I woke up from the sleeping med, and I was told by the doctor, that the test showed that I had four bleeding ulcers, and this truly freaked me out, I had heard of ulcer before, but I didn't know that you can have more than one., what I did know is, that I never had ulcer issues during my ten year run with hemo. I never really knew what caused these ulcers. I have been on a medication for almost a decade now, I am OK taking this medicine, but I can't eat grapefruit anymore, in which I have loved to eat, especially for breakfast. Now, I am turning 50, and of course, it is mandatory that if you want to be still considerate for a cadaver kidney, a patient has to have a colonoscopy, to continue being a candidate for a cadaver kidney, well I had the colonoscopy, but it wasn't as easy for me to get prepared for the colonoscopy, because there was a pre-prepping diet, that I had to follow. Now mind you, I am a PD patient, that has to dwell an excessive amount of fluid (solution) in my peritoneum. Let me break it down to you, the scenarios around my prepping for the procedure.

Storing of peritoneal dialysis supplies:

When storing PD supplies, first, they shouldn't ever be stored in the garage, because of potential dampness. I am fortunate to have space, under the stairs of my home, to store most of my supplies, and those large boxes of solution. The manual bags, come eight bags in a box, which range from

1000 bags to 2000 bags, and the cycler bags are much larger, and they come two to a box, which my bags are 6000ML bags. I place most of my boxes against a wall, one side for manuals and other side for cycler bags. And I have shelves to house, the various other supplies, such as gloves, mask, mini-caps, tape, betadine, alcohol preps, syringes, and IV gauges. I also keep a small supply for about a week usage, upstairs in my bedroom, also a couple of boxes of manuals, and cycler boxes are also kept upstairs. All in all, you have to make room for an excessive amount of supplies for PD. With the order of the supplies, in the beginning your PD nurse will do the ordering, and after you have started manual PD, she will teach you to start ordering your own supplies. The most important thing, is to never run out, just keep tabs on the amount of boxes, that you have on hand, although there have been incidences where I ran out of a certain solution, and most cases, you can get some from your home unit, until you receive your emergency supply, or if it is time to do your inventory to reorder supplies. There was a time, when I ran out of 1.5, because I used a great deal of it, while in the hospital, because the hospital didn't supply my particular ML they only supplied the standard 2500ML bags, and I can't dwell that much fill volume, well anyway, I tried to get some from my home unit, but they were fresh out, and I had to wait for my emergency supply, so I was forced to do all manual exchanges, which meant, I would run out of my manual bags at some point. Yes, it can be frustrating at times, when it comes to the supplies. Just keep a close eye on your supplies at all times, and most importantly, doing any changes in your particular prescription.

Keeping my PD catherer safe, is very important, so when I first started dialysis, I was concerned if the seatbelt would be harmful to my catherer, so I place a small pillow over my catherer, before I fasten my seatbelt. When I went out to purchase a small pillow, I couldn't find one, so I saw a small pillow in my little great nieces bedroom, and I thought to myself, I know where I can get one of those small pillows from, so I visit the kids R us store, and purchase one of the kiddy pillows, I also acquired a small pillow, when I took a trip, and the airline provided those little small pillows, that I kept, and that is another pillow that works for me. Just wanted to share this little tip with you PD patients.

Preparation for Colonscopy Procedure: On Peritoneal Dialysis

First, I was told, that I needed to stop my aggrenox (a medication that I was prescribed after my second minor stroke). I discuss this with my primary dr., and she said in her opinion, that stopping the aggrenox, five days before the procedure, could be a risk of developing another stroke, so she left it up to me, to decide to stop the med for that time. I truly would like to be considered for a transplant, so that was my only decision to make. I stopped the meds, as instructed. Now, on with the days of pre-prepping for the procedure.

7 days - prior to colonoscopy - Colyte Prep

First stop the aggrenox - also avoid all aspirin or aspirin containing products - such as: motrin, Excedrin and Iron.

3 days - prior to colonoscopy - follow low fiber diet
Instructions - Milk and milk products - can be eaten, but in the case of a dialysis patient having this procedure, please avoid all milk products - phosphorus alert!

Group	Can Eat	Avoid
Vegetables	green beans	vegetable juice w/pulp
	Wax beans	and raw vegetables
	Spinach	
	Pumpkin	
	Eggplant	
	Potatoes without skin	
	Asparagus	
	Beets	
	Carrots	

Fruits	Fruit juice w/o pulp Ripe bananas, and all Canned fruit except Pineapple	Fruit juices with pulp, canned pineapple, and fresh fruit
Starches- Bread And Grains	Bread and cereal made from refined flours (white) Pasta, and white rice	whole-grain breads and cereals, oatmeal, brown rice and pasta
Meat or Meat Substitute	Meat, poultry, eggs and Seafood	Chunky peanut butter, nuts, seeds, dried beans
Fats and Oils	All oils, margarine and Butter	None
Sweets and Desserts	All not on avoid list	Desserts containing nuts or Coconut
Miscellaneous	All not on avoid list	Popcorn, pickles, relish

This is the low fiber selection that I made: Note: the list is limited
For breakfast - I had one pouched egg, 1 cup of orange juice w/o pulp, and slice of white toast.

For Lunch - I had baked talipia (fish), recipe - I took four talipia filets, and seasoned with a sprinkle of a mixture, of a dash of tarragon, creole seasoning, onion powder, garlic powder and Mrs. Dash table blend, placed this fish in a glass casserole dish, and poured 1 ¼ cup of chicken broth over it, with a dash of ½ tsp. Worchestire sauce, and ½ tsp. Rice wine vinegar. Bake at 350 degrees, for about 20 minutes, depending on your oven. Mashed potatoes with out the skin, about four stalks of steamed asparagus, and ½ glass of ginger ale.

For Dinner - Broiled chicken breast, ½ cup of steamed green beans, one slice of white bread, and ½ cup of apple juice.
Note: I followed this menu for two days

Day before Colonoscopy:

Follow a Clear Liquid Diet: It is very important to follow the clear liquid diet, because clear liquids supply fluids and energy from foods that need very little digestion. These fluids contain certain salts and minerals, which help in preventing dehydration. The value of the examination will depend on getting a thoroughly clean bowel.

At 10:00 a.m. - I took 2 ducolax (stool softeners) w/water, I then pre-mixed the Colyte w/crystal light, so that it will have a better taste, (but you can use water, if you prefer) - per the instructions - and stored in the refrigerator.

1:00 p.m. - 2:00 p.m. - I drinked 8 ozs. - every 10 - 15 minutes, it took me about 4 hours to finish this Colyte, I immediately drinked an additional 64 ounces of chicken broth, and drink the broth in two hour. Now, because I am on PD, I learned something during one of my hospital stays, when a CT Scan was ordered, with the CT Scan, I had to drink a liquid substance, to prepare for the CT Scan, but at the time, when I would tried to drink this required liquid, I would throw it up, so I realized, that the PD solution that was dwelling in my stomach, wasn't allowing the liquid substance to stay down. I immediately brought this to the attention of the nurse, and she told me to drain half of the PD solution, and it worked, I was able to keep the liquid down, so this incident at the hospital, prompted me to use this very same strategy, when it came to drinking this Colyte, to prepare for the colonoscopy procedure. So, anyone, that may have the same situation as I do, with the PD solution, and having to drink this Colyte for a colonoscopy, try filling only half of your PD solution for dwelling, and it would be advisable to do all manual exchanges during this preparation stage for the colonoscopy.

I continued to drink clear liquids until midnight, such as tea, water, and broth, and nothing else to eat or drink, until after the colonoscopy is done.

My procedure was scheduled for 9:30 a.m., and I needed to be there at 8:30 a.m., when I arrived, I checked in, and had to sign a consent form for the procedure. I was provided a gown and told to undress from the waist down and remove any long sleeved garments. I was then placed on a gurney. The nurse came in to insert an intravenous (IV) line for the administering of fluids/sedating medications of such, she then applied the monitoring equipment and then the nurse made sure, that all the paperwork was completed and signed. This process took about 20 minutes. The physician then came in, and evaluated me, and it was applicable, he also explained to me, how the procedure is done, and why it is being done. He insures me that the colonoscopy is a very useful diagnostic examination, which is the most accurate way of examining the colon to detect and remove abnormalities like polyps, and I asked him what are polyps?, and he responds, by saying, polyps are abnormal growths of tissue, which can vary in size from 1/8 to an inch or more. He also said polyps, are slow growing, but may cause rectal bleeding and may develop into colon cancer. He also told me what will be done, he said a flexible video instrument (called a colon scope) will be inserted through the rectum and advanced through the entire colon. All this sound very devastating to me, but he assured me, that it is a very painless procedure, that most don't even remember anything about the procedure, after it is completed, and that is when he sedated me for the procedure with a sedative along with a narcotic pain medication. I must have went to sleep, because when I woke up, I was in recovery, and the nurse, summoned the physician, and he came in, and said congratulations, there are no polyps or masses identified, but you do have Diverticulosis, but it is mild on the left side. He did give me some instructions, to follow a high fiber diet, and to avoid seeded food as much as possible, because of the diverticulosis. He then gave me a print out of my colon with description of the findings and results. Of course, with my very curious mind, I wanted to know what was diverticulosis, and he responded by explaining it to me, they are small pouches in your colon, that bulge outward through weak spots, like an inner tube that pokes through weak places in a tire, and each pouch is called a diverticulum when the pouches become infected or inflamed, the condition is called diverticulitis. The physician also informed me, that there is a increased risk of diverticulitis in poly cystic kidney disease patients. After talking with the doctor, I was allowed to go home. It was mandatory, that my husband be there, while I was having the procedure, and to also drive me home.

Issues with Dialysis

Through my 20 years of dialysis treatment, with both Hemo dialysis and Peritoneal Dialysis, I have had my issues with my appearance. First, lets touch base with my phosphorus issues. It took a few years, for me to finally understand the importance of keeping the phosphorus in normal range, as best as I can, but of course, that is easier said than done. During my early days of hemo, I was having problems with uncontrollable itching. I would use a anti-itch lotion (OTC), to relieve the itching, but this only brings temporary relief. At the time, I was prescribed calcium phosphate, but this med, wasn't binding my phosphorus very well, because I was still having these darn itching attacks, I would be irritable on varies parts of my body, especially my arms and legs. The scratching would leave scars. I tried using a back scratcher, per a fellow patient's advice, but this also only relieve me temporary. While I was having treatment, I began to have itching, and I was administered benadryl, to relieve the itching, I guess the nurse, didn't want a patient scratching, because they may move around too much, during the treatment, and cause unnecessary alarms to go off. The only thing with benadryl, is the fact that it makes me very sleepy. It wasn't a good thing for me to be administered benadryl, because most times it didn't wear off, by time, my treatment was over, because of the fact, that I drove myself to the unit, most of the time. My neprologist prescribed benadryl for me to take by mouth, when needed for itching. I didn't want to rely on benadryl so often for relief, so I took it upon myself, to learn as much about phosphorus, as I can. I did learn that I needed to limit the phosphorus in my renal diet, and to always take phosphorus binders to help in binding this mineral, before it could reach my bloodstream. Phosphorus is a mineral that works together with calcium to keep the bones strong and healthy, but people with kidney disease, have to be careful with their diet, because their kidneys won't get rid of this extra phosphorus, like normal functioning kidneys do. And I learned that if I continue to eat high phosphorus foods and neglect to take my binders, I will start to experience uncontrollable itching (in which I did), and if it continues to be neglected, my bones could get brittle, I could get hardening of the blood vessels and body organs, which could lead to a heart attack, and the potential for renal bone disease and calcifications in soft tissues, (such as - the hearts and lungs). I could also have pain in my bones and joints, and of course red eyes. I could also get calcification in my eyes, foot, etc., I saw a display of this calcification at my unit a few years ago, and it was so hideous, Wow! It truly scared me, to the point, that ever since seeing this display, I have been trying my best to watch my phosphorus intake and to always take my binders. I have this rule, Eat, Bind, Drink, Bind.

Such foods as: Ice Cream, Cream Soups, Chowders, Peanut Butter, Whole Wheat Bread, Chocolate, and Dark Sodas like - Coke Cola, Pepsi, and Dr. Pepper, should be limited as much as possible. I haven't eaten Ice Cream, Peanut Butter, Whole Wheat Bread, Chocolate, and all dark sodas in over fifteen years. It was very hard for me in the beginning to just stop eating Ice Cream. I substitute the Ice Cream, for Italian Ice, and I am OK with that, because I adore Italian Ice. I don't even miss or crave Ice Cream anymore. I know there was a time in the beginning that I couldn't stand seeing anyone eating Ice Cream, but it doesn't bother me at all anymore. I know I have the determination and the will, to ignore these indulges. I don't know the last time, I had a piece of chocolate of any kind, and that doesn't bother me in the least, anymore. My dietitian suggested that I consider drinking the lite drinks, such as 7-Up, Ginger Ale, Sprite, or Sierra Mist. I was even urged to limit my intake of Hawaiian Punch, in which I have always loved. However, I do take my binders, but I had to make some changes to my binder regiment, because for some reason they weren't working for me. My dietitian and I came to the conclusion that, because I am a slow eater, that I shouldn't take all my binders at once, my regiment is five with meals, and three with snacks. I decided to take three at the beginning of my meal, and two more towards the end of my meal, and it has worked out very well for me. I don't have any more elevated levels of phosphorus, but on occasion, it is right on the cuff of the end of the normal range, and believe it or not, it is sometimes on the low end. Which the normal range for phosphorus is 3.5 -5.5 mg.

Now, let me share with you some of the foods, that I eat, and how much phosphorus these foods contain.

When it comes to dairy products, they tend to have an excessive amount of phosphorus

Check out these dairy products and how much phosphorus they contain.

150 mg - the low category of phosphorus foods, such as:

Butter - 1 tbsp - 3 mg

Cheese - brie - 1 oz - 53mg

Cheese - feta - 1 oz. - 96mg

Cottage cheese - nonfat - ½ cup - 76mg

Cream cheese - 1 oz. - 30 mg

Cream - half & half - 1 tbsp - 14mg

Egg white - 1 med. - 4mg

Egg yolk - 1 med. - 86mg

Ice Cream - 10% -
vanilla - ½ cup - 67mg

Sherbert - ½ cup - 38mg

Sour cream - ½ cup - 98mg

151 to 200 mg - the higher (moderate) category of phosphorus foods, such as:

Cheese, blue - 1 oz - 110 mg

Cheese, cheddar - 1 oz - 145 mg

Cheese, mozzarella - 1 oz - 105 mg

Cheese, provolone - 1 oz - 141 mg

Cheese, Swiss - 1 oz - 171 mg

Cottage Cheese - 4% fat - ½ cup - 139 mg

Cottage Cheese - 2% fat - ½ cup - 170 mg

Ice milk, soft serve, vanilla - ½ cup - 106 mg

201 mg or more - the highest category of phosphorus foods, such as:

Buttermilk, 1 cup - 219 mg

Cheese, parmesan - 1 oz - 229 mg

Cheese, ricotta, part skim - ½ cup - 226 mg

Milk, evaporated skim - ½ cup - 248 mg

Milk, nonfat - 1 cup - 247-275 mg (depending on the brand)

Milk, whole - 1 cup - 228 mg

Processed American cheese - 1 oz - 211 mg

Legumes (beans) - something I grew up on, and big pots of it, but since starting dialysis, I had to limit the amount that I consume in my renal diet: these nutritional facts are based on a ½ cup serving - cooked and these fall in the low category of phosphorus - to 100 mg

Peas, split - 97 mg

Peanuts - boiled - 63 mg

Soy milk - 59 mg

101 to 150 mg - higher (moderate) category of phosphorus:

Black beans - 120 mg
Kidney beans - 125 mg
Lima beans - (thick) - 104 mg   based on a ½ cup serving - cooked
Lima beans - (thin) - 116 mg
Navy beans - 143 mg
Pinto beans - 146 mg
Black-eyed peas - 134 mg
Chickpeas - 137 mg

151 or more mg - highest category of phosphorus - based on a ½ cup serving - cooked

White beans - (small) - 152 mg   Soybeans - 211 mg
Lentils - 176 mg

Now, when it comes to Seafood, which usually is very healthy for you, but when the kidneys function has diminished, the phosphorus contain in the seafood is in question, with the renal diet. Being born and raised in the south, I grew up on a great deal of seafood. My mom would prepare it at least once a week. Here is a breakdown of how much phosphorus is in some of my favorite seafood - these nutritional facts are based on a 3 oz serving cooked or as stated:

To 150 mg - low category of phosphorus:
Based on a 3 oz serving

Clams - 144 mg   Oysters, pacific, raw - 136mg
Cod, atlantic - 117 mg   Shrimp - boiled - 116mg

151 to 200 mg - higher category of phosphorus:

Catfish, breaded, or fried - 183 mg
Crab, blue, moist heat - 175 mg
Crab, Dungeness, moist heat - 149 mg
Cod, pacific - 190 mg   **(based on 3 oz serving -**
Lobster, moist heat - 157 mg   **dry/cooked or as stated)**
Mussels, blue, raw - 168 mg
Shrimp, breaded or fried - 185 mg
Shrimp, canned - 198 mg
Red snapper - 171 mg

Tuna, light, canned in water - 158 mg

201 or more mg - highest category of phosphorus:
Calamari, fried - 213 mg
Clams, moist heat - 287 mg
Crab, Alaskan, moist heat - 238 mg
Flounder - 246 mg
Halibut - 242 mg
Oysters, Eastern, cooked - 236 mg   **(based on 3 oz serving - dry/**
Mussels, blue, cooked - 242 mg   **cooked or as stated)**
Salmon, canned, pink/red - 279 mg
Salmon, fresh, cooked - 234 mg
Scallops, breaded, fried - 203 mg
Filet of sole - 246 mg
Tuna, white, canned in oil - 227 mg
Tuna, light, in oil - 265 mg

For your information: some Grains and Cereals - need to be limit in the renal diet also, here is a breakdown of nutritional facts, that pertain to the amount of phosphorus contained in a variety of Grains and Cereals - Portions as stated:

To 65 mg - low category of phosphorus foods:
Bagel, plain - 3 ½" diameter - one - 46 mg
Barley, pearled, cooked - ½ cup - 43 mg
Bread, pita, 6 ½ " diameter - one - 60 mg   **(portions as stated)**
Bread, white - 1 slice - 27 mg
Corn flakes, plain - 1 cup - 14 mg
Couscous, cooked - ½ cup - 20 mg
Crispy rice cereal - 1 cup - 31mg
Farina, cooked - ¾ cup - 21 mg
Hominy grits - ½ cup - 15 mg
Rice, white, cooked - ½ cup - 37 mg

65 to 150 mg - higher category of phosphorus foods:
Bread, pumpernickel, 1 slice - 71 mg
Bread, whole wheat - 1 slice - 66 mg
English, muffin, plain - one - 67 mg
Oatmeal, cooked - 1 packet - 133 mg   **(portions as stated)**

Pasta, "al dente" - 1 cup - 85 mg
Raisin Bran, ½ cup - 124 mg
Rice, brown, cooked - ½ cup - 81 mg
Shredded wheat, 1 large biscuit - 86 mg
Wheat flakes - 1 cup - 100 mg
Wheat flour, white, 1 cup - 135 mg

151 or more mg - highest category of phosphorus foods:
Note: these foods should be limited as much as possible in the renal diet

Bran cereal, 100% - ½ cup - 402 mg
Corn flour, whole grain - 1 cup - 318 mg   **(portions as stated)**
Cornmeal, whole grain - 1 cup - 294 mg
Wheat flour, whole grain - 1 cup - 415 mg
Wheat germ, plain, toasted - ¼ cup - 324 mg

SNACKS - There are some snacks that contain an excessive amount of phosphorus, which should be limited also in the renal diet and always take your binders, as prescribed for snacks, it is usually least taken than a actual meal.

To 65 mg - lowest category of phosphorus foods:
Chestnuts, Chinese style, canned, 2 oz - 10 mg   **(portions as stated)**
Cookies, shortbread, 4 small - 39 mg
Gelatin, water base, ½ cup - 23 mg - Note: this is also counted as fluid intake count
Popcorn, air popped - 1 cup - 22 mg
Rice cake - one - 34 mg
Cool whip - 2 tbsp - 0 mg

66 to 150 mg - higher category of phosphorus foods:
Angel food cake - 1/12 - 91 mg
Cocoa, dry, unsweetened - 2 tbsp - 74 mg   **(portions as stated)**
Macadamia nuts, oil roasted - 2 oz - 114 mg

151 mg - highest category of phosphorus foods:
Note: these high phosphorus foods, should be limited as much as possible in the renal diet

Almonds, oil/dry roasted - 2 oz - 312 mg
Cashews, dry roasted - 2 oz - 278 mg
Cashews, oil roasted - 2 oz - 242 mg   **(portions as stated)**
Pecans, oil/dry roasted - 2 oz - 170 mg
Walnuts, black - 2 oz - 264 mg
Walnuts, English - 2oz - 180 mg

Meat - yes, there are meats that contain an excessive amount of phosphorus:
To 150 mg - lowest category of phosphorus foods:
Beef, ground, extra lean - 137 mg
Beef, ground, regular - 144 mg **Based on 3 oz serving - dry/cooked**
Duck, domestic, with skin on - 133 mg

151 to 200 mg - higher category of phosphorus foods:
Beef, chuck roast - 163 mg
Beef, eye round - 177 mg
Beef, sirloin steak - 186 mg   **Based on a 3 oz -**
Chicken, white - 185 mg   **serving - dry/cooked**
Chicken, dark - 154 mg
Lamb, kabobs, domestic - 190 mg   **(Note: there are a variety of**
Lamb, leg roast, domestic - 162 mg   **lamb, and the phosphorus**
Lamb, leg roast, New Zealand - 186 mg **content varies)**

Pork, fresh, loin ribs - 142 mg
Turkey, white - 188 mg
Turkey, dark - 157 mg

201 or more mg - highest category of phosphorus foods:
Again, it is advisable to limit these foods, as much as possible in the renal diet
Beef, bottom round - 217 mg
Beefalo - 213 mg
Pork, fresh, boneless loin chop - 203 mg   **Based on a 3 oz - serving**
Pork, fresh, leg roast - 224 mg   **- dry/cooked**
Pork, fresh, spareribs - 192 mg
Veal, cubes, stewed - 203 mg
Veal, rib roast - 211 mg

Potassium - is an important mineral, that needs to be monitored, when it comes to a renal diet:

I can relate to both the high and low sector of potassium, during my ten year run with hemo, I had the difficult task of limiting the potassium in my diet, because my potassium levels tend to fall in the high level, and of course, just about everything you eat, has some form of potassium in its contents, and I will share with you some of the low, higher, and highest category of potassium food:

A little education is in order, to help you to understand the importance of keeping the potassium in normal range, especially in the process of keeping your heart happy. (Smile)
Potassium is a mineral just like sodium, that is essential for your body. Its purpose is to help regulate muscle contractions. The most important muscle being the **HEART.** Now, too much or too little *potassium in* your blood can cause your heart to beat irregular and it can possibly stop beating. A high potassium level can be life-threatening.

When the kidneys are functioning normally, they regulate the blood level of potassium in your body for you, but when your kidneys are not functioning, you must control your potassium level by the foods that you eat. The potassium level in your bloodstream may rise very quickly and can occur without warning signs or symptoms, however, if you feel lethargic, tingling of extremities, muscle weakness, irritable or confused, **PLEASE CALL YOUR DOCTOR OR DIALYSIS UNIT!**

Although potassium is found in all foods, we must learn to avoid the foods that are particularly high in potassium. There are certain fruits and vegetables that are very high in potassium, and if you have issues with high potassium in your body, it is your job to learn which fruits and vegetable are the trouble makers of potassium.

Important facts about potassium: Potassium is water soluble, this means that if you cook a vegetable like carrots, (for instance) - in a large amount of water, some of the potassium will leave the vegetable and deposit in the water. So a carrot cooked in water is lower in potassium, than a raw carrot. Mashed potatoes are lower in potassium than a baked potato. As a general rule of thumb, frozen and canned vegetables, as well as fruit, are lower in potassium than fresh vegetables and fruits.

Potassium is also accumulative, which means that even though a fruit or vegetable have low potassium, if you eat a large quantity, it will add up. For example: take cherries (for instance), if you eat maybe a handful, it could still keep your potassium levels low, but eating two pounds of cherries in one sitting is way too much. Spreading out your potassium intake throughout the day, you can better monitor, how much you maybe consuming in one single day.

Beware, of salt substitute, even though they maybe low in sodium, you have to be careful of the potassium chloride, in its content, also lite salt and low sodium bouillon cubes, have an excessive amount of potassium in its content.

Here is a list of some of the potassium foods, and the mg they contain of potassium

To 150 mg - Low category of Potassium
From 151 - 200 mg - Higher category of Potassium
201 mg or more mg - Highest category of Potassium

Beverages - based on a ½ cup serving
Apple juice - ½ cup - 148 mg
Coffee - 6 oz - brewed - 124 mg
Cranberry juice - ½ cup - 31 mg
Ginger ale - 12 oz - 4 mg
Tea, 6 oz - brewed - 27 mg

Low category of potassium - To 120 mg - based on a ½ cup serving, raw
Apples, peeled, sliced - 62 mg
Applesauce, canned, sweetened - 78 mg; unsweetened - 92 mg
Apricot, 1 medium - 105 mg
Blueberries, raw - 65 mg
Cherries, sour, red canned, water packed - 120 mg
Cranberries, raw - 39 mg

Cranberry sauce, canned, sweetened - 36 mg
Fig, fresh - 1 medium - 116 mg
Fruit cocktail, canned, heavy syrup - 112 mg; juice pack - 118 mg
Grape, Thompson seedless - ten (10) - 93 mg
Grapes, Tokay, Emperor seeded, ten (10) - 105 mg
Lemon, 1 medium - 80 mg
Lime, 1 medium - 68 mg
Peaches, canned, heavy syrup - 118 mg
Pears, cooked, heavy syrup - 83 mg; juice pack - 119 mg
Pineapple, raw, diced - 88 mg
Plums, canned, heavy syrup - 118 mg
Plums, raw - 1 medium - 114 mg
Raspberries - raw - 94 mg
Rhubarb, cooked, with sugar - 115 mg
Watermelon - diced - ½ cup - 93 mg

Higher category of potassium - 121 to 250 mg - based on ½ cup serving or otherwise stated:
Apricots, canned, heavy syrup - 181 mg; juice packed - 205 mg
Blackberries, raw - 141 mg
Cherries, sweet - ten (10) - 152 mg
Elderberries, raw - 203 mg
Grapefruit - ½ medium - 167 mg
Grapefruit - canned, with syrup - 164 mg
Orange - 1 medium - 237 mg
Peach, 1 medium - 171 mg
Peaches, canned, juice packed - 159 mg
Pear, Asian - 1 medium - 148 mg
Pear - 1 medium - Bosc - 176 mg; Bartlett - 208 mg; D'Anjou - 250 mg
Pineapple, canned, pieces; heavy syrup - 133 mg
Pineapple, caned, pieces, juice packed - 153 mg
Plums, canned, juice packed - 194 mg
Prickly pear - 1 medium - 226 mg
Raspberries, frozen, sweetened - 143 mg
Strawberries, raw - 124 mg
Strawberries, frozen, sweetened, sliced - 125 mg
Tangerine - 1 medium - 132 mg

Highest category of potassium - 251 or more mg

Apricots, dried, uncooked - 896 mg

Apricots, dried, cooked, unsweetened & liquid - 611mg

Avocado, ½ medium - California - 549 mg; Florida - 742 mg

Banana - medium - 451 mg

Cantaloupe - ¼ medium - 413 mg

Dates - chopped - 581 mg

Figs - five (5) - dried - 666 mg

Honeydew Melon - ¼ medium - 875 mg

Kiwifruit - 1 medium - 252 mg

Mango - 1 medium - 323 mg

Nectarine - 1 medium - 288 mg

Papaya - ½ medium - 390 mg

Peaches - dried, cooked, unsweetened and liquid - 413 mg

Peaches - dried, uncooked - 797 mg

Plantain, boiled or sliced - 358 mg

Pomegranate - 1 medium - 399 mg

Prunes - cooked, unsweetened & liquid - 354 mg

Prunes - five (5) - dried, uncooked - 365 mg

Raisins, seedless - 545 mg

Sapodilla - 1 medium - 328 mg

Vegetables & Starches - based on ½ cup serving or as stated:
Lowest category of potassium - To 125 mg

Alfalfa seeds - sprouted, raw, - 13 mg

Arugula, raw - 37 mg

Bagel, plain - 50 mg

Bamboo shoots, canned - 53 mg

Beans, green, cooked from frozen - 76 mg

Bean sprout, raw - 78 mg

Bean sprout, cooked - 63 mg

Bread - one slice - white - 28 mg

Cabbage - raw, red - 72; common - 86 mg

Carrots, cooked from frozen - 116 mg

Cauliflower, cooked from frozen - 125 mg

Collards, leaves, cooked from raw - 84 mg

Corn, cooked from frozen - 114 mg

Cucumbers, sliced - 84 mg

Dandelion greens, cooked - 121 mg
Eggplant, steamed - 119 mg
Endive, raw - 79 mg
Jicama, raw - 98 mg
Leeks, cooked from raw - 46 mg; raw - 94 mg
Lettuce, iceberg - 1 cup - 87 mg
Mustard greens, cooked from frozen - 104 mg
Oatmeal, regular - ¾ cup - 99 mg
Onions, raw, diced - 124 mg
Pasta, plain "al dente" - 1 cup - 103 mg
Peppers, sweet, raw - 89 mg
Popcorn, air popped - 1 cup - 20 mg
Radicchio, raw, shredded - 60 mg
Rice, cooked, white - 29; brown - 69 mg
Turnips, white, cubes, cooked from raw - 106 mg
Water chestnuts, canned - 83 mg

Higher category of potassium - 126 to 250 mg - based on ½ cup serving or as stated:
Asparagus, cooked from frozen - 196 mg
Beans, green, cooked from raw - 185 mg
Bread, pumpernickel, 1 slice - 141 mg
Broccoli, cooked from frozen - 167 mg
Broccoli, cooked from raw - 127 mg
Brussels sprouts, cooked from raw - 246 mg
Cabbage, common, cooked - 154 mg
Carrots, cooked from raw - 177 mg
Carrots, raw, grated - 178 mg
Cauliflower, cooked from raw - 202 mg
Cauliflower, raw, florets - 178 mg
Celery, raw, diced - 171 mg
Chickpeas, cooked, drained - 239 mg
Collards, cooked from frozen - 214 mg
Corn, cooked from raw - 204 mg
Fennel bulb, raw, sliced - 180 mg
Kale, cooked from frozen - 209 mg
Kale, cooked from raw - 148 mg
Lettuce, romaine - 1 cup - 148 mg

Mushrooms, raw - 130 mg
Mustard Greens, cooked from raw - 141 mg
Okra, sliced, cooked from frozen - 215 mg
Onions, cooked - 160 mg
Parsley, raw - 166 mg
Peas, edible pod, cooked - 192 mg
Peas, green, cooked from frozen - 134 mg
Peppers, hot chili, 1 raw - 153 mg
Radishes, raw - 144 mg
Scallions, raw - 138 mg
Squash, summer, cooked - (all types) - 173 mg
Spinach, raw, chopped - 154 mg
Tomatillos, raw - chopped - 177 mg
Tortillas, corn flour - 172 mg
Turnip greens, cooked from frozen - 184 mg
Turnip greens, cooked from raw - 146 mg
Turnips, white, cubes, cooked from frozen - 142 mg

Highest category of potassium - 251 mg or more mg - based on a ½ cup serving or as stated:
Artichoke - 1 medium - 425 mg
Asparagus, cooked from raw - 279 mg
Beet greens, cooked - 654 mg
Beets, cooked, diced or sliced - 265 mg
Cabbage, bok choi - cooked - 316 mg
Kohlrabi, cooked - 281 mg
Lettuce, Boston, one 5" head - 419 mg
Lentils, cooked - 366 mg
Mushrooms, cooked - 278 mg
Okra, sliced, cooked from raw - 257 mg
Parsnips, cooked - 287 mg
Peanuts, oil roasted, unsalted - 491 mg
Peas, split, cooked - 355 mg
Potato, baked - 1 large - (no skin) - 610 mg
Potato, baked - 1 large - (with skin) - 844 mg
Potatoes, boiled - (no skin) - 256 mg
Pumpkin, canned - 253 mg
Pumpkin, cooked from raw - 282 mg

Rutabagas, cubes, cooked - 277 mg
Soybeans, cooked - 486 mg
Spinach, cooked from frozen - 283 mg
Spinach, cooked from raw - 420 mg
Squash, winter, cooked - (all types) - 448 mg
Sweet potato - 1 medium - baked - 397 mg
Sweet potato - ½ cup - peeled, boiled - 301 mg
Tomato, raw - 1 medium - green - 251 mg
Tomato, raw - 1 medium - red - 273 mg

I have had other personal health issues through the years. During my ten year run with hemo dialysis, I experienced severe swelling of the body. All this came about after a bout with my first transplant experience, having a subclavian (catherer), that wasn't a successful surgical procedure, which after losing the transplanted kidney, after four months of normal function, returning to hemo, edema became a very serious issue. I had a great deal of compromising, when it came to my wardrobe, my swelling was so severe, that I could no longer fit most of my wardrobe. Thank God, for Ross Retail Outlet, I was able to buy some clothes, that fit comfortably, and most importantly, very affordable. I also resulted to slip on footwear, like clogs and slipper type shoes. It was so strange to me, because my body was swelling more on the left side, and that happen to be the side of the neck, where I had this very blotched up catherer surgically placed. Although after that, I also had issues about four months after starting hemo dialysis, I noticed that my foundation had all of a sudden become too light for my face, it seemed that the dialysis treatment was changing my complexion, I became a couple shades darker. I had to change my foundation to a much darker shade. And the trip thing with this was, A couple of months, after receiving the blessing of a cadaver kidney, I noticed my foundation became too dark for my face. I was once again, changing my foundation to a much lighter shade. Now after this issue was resolved, my period stopped after six months of dialysis, as soon as I received the blessing of a cadaver kidney, my period came back full force, this simply amazed me, because I had to go out and buy some sanitary protection, ain't that something. So much drama, so much issues. Now, in my 10th year of peritoneal dialysis, yes, I have my personal issues with PD. First, I am a very small framed person, and being on peritoneal dialysis, has its disadvantages, my appearance for one thing, my stomach bulges out, and it appears like I am about five months pregnant, of course, this was devastating to me in the beginning, but I soon adjusted to it, and find a little compromise, where my wardrobe was concerned, I began to wear large size tops, which I found some very fashionable large tops. I could no longer wear belts around my waist, and the tops had to be long enough to cover over my bulging stomach. At least my PD scar didn't have to be visible, but I did have some very large scars on my arms from grafts. They became the center of conversation, and there was an occasion, I was mistaken for a drug addict, because of the needle markings that were quite visible on my arms, and of course, these marks were also mistaken for gun shot wounds. I remember this one time, when I was visiting a friend of mine, and her kids immediately thought I had been shot, the trip thing is, they didn't ask me had I been shot, they had the nerve to ask me who shot me. They innocently ask this, because of what they had seen in their neighborhood on a regular basis, especially living in this type of environment, with drug pushers and prostitutes living and roaming in their neighborhood. I just tried to explain to them, that the scars were from a medical treatment I had to have to stay alive. I am sure they didn't understand, but I did ease their concerns about my numerous scars I had to endure, because of these treatments. I had just finished my dialysis treatment, and decided to drove to the Pacific Telephone Company to pay my bill, and while I was waiting in that seemly long endless line, I became very faint, and I immediately set on the floor against the wall, because I remembered when my blood pressure would plummeted at the unit, the nurse would practically recline my chair almost to the floor. As I was sitting in an Indian sit (beside the wall), two toddler kids sat down right beside me, and thought I wanted to play with them, and that is when those kids mom, was whispering to someone else in line, that she ain't nothing but a drug addict, trying to pay a bill, and high off, I don't know what, and the other lady customer, that she was talking to, ask why do you think that, well look at her arm, its loaded with needle tracks. At that moment, I was too weak, to respond to her, but I was very angry at her insinuation. These were some of the personal issues that I was faced with, because people weren't educated about kidney disease and dialysis, but it is a little more known today. People today, either know someone or have a loved one surviving with the blessing of dialysis. And it is a blessing, well to me, because there was a time some fifty years ago, when there wasn't any such treatment, for people with kidney disease, to live a somewhat normal life.

Also, experiencing two minor strokes, in the last decade, I realized how important it is to keep the blood pressure under control, because of my erratic blood pressure, high as well as low at times, I developed a stroke, from this see saw blood pressure. After the second stroke, I began to research strokes, and I do remember the struggle that my Grandma Martha had when she had a major stroke (back in the early 1960's, when there wasn't enough education on a stroke), which left her paralyzed on her left side, and she also lost the ability to speak. Because of the second stroke, my insurance company was kind enough to send me some literature, that will help me to understand why a stroke could occur and ways of how to prevent a future stroke from occurring, and I would like to share this literature with my readers.

What is a stroke?
A stroke is damage to part of the brain, when its blood supply is suddenly reduced or stopped. A stroke may also be called a cerebral vascular accident, or CVA. The part of the brain deprived of blood dies and can no longer function.

How does a stroke occur?
Blood is prevented from reaching brain tissue when a blood vessel leading to the brain becomes blocked or bursts (hemorrhagic).

Factors that have the potential to increase the risk of a stroke:

* high blood pressure
* diabetes
* high cholesterol level
* cigarette smoking
* being overweight
* family history of stroke
* heart valve or heart muscle disease called endocarditic
* hardening of the arteries (fatty cholesterol deposits on artery walls, atherosclerosis)
* heart disease or coronary artery disease)
* heart rhythm problems such as arterial fibrillation
* sleep apnea
* sickle cell anemia
* cocaine use

* Triglycerides blood level of 150 mg/dl or more
* HDL cholesterol levels below 40 mg/dl for men and below 50 mg/dl for women
* blood pressure of 130/85 mm HG or higher
* predicaments (a fasting blood sugar between 100 and 125) or diabetes (a fasting blood sugar level over 125 mg/dl)
* and believe or not, excessive weight around the waist (waist measurement of more Than 40 inches for men and more than 35 inches for women)

Possible symptoms of a stroke:
Note: the symptoms of a stroke differ, depending on the part of the brain affected and the extent of the damage. Symptoms following a stroke come on suddenly and may include:

* weakness, numbness, or tingling in the face, arm, or leg, especially on one side of the body
* trouble walking, dizziness, loss of balance, or coordination
* inability to speak or difficulty speaking or understanding
* trouble seeing with one or both eyes, or double vision
* difficulty with muscle movements, such as swallowing, moving arms and legs
* lost of bowel and bladder control
* severe headache with no known causes
* loss of consciousness

Warnings known as transient ischemic attacks (TIAs) may happen before the actual stroke. TIAs occur when the blood supply to the brain is reduced for a short time without causing permanent damage. A TIA is sometimes referred to as a mini-stroke, because it causes the same symptoms as a stroke, but the symptoms go away within minutes to a few hours. It is very important to call **911**, if you see or experience any of these symptoms. Treatment can be more effective if given quickly, because every minute counts.

How is it diagnosed?
If symptoms of a stroke occur, someone should call an ambulance or take you to an emergency room right away.

Your healthcare provider will know from your symptoms and physical exam whether you are having a stroke.

The following tests may be done:

* blood tests
* brain scan, such as a CT scan or MRI
* carotid ultrasound to look at blood flow in the carotid arteries in the neck
* cerebral arteriolar to look at the blood vessels in the brain
* electrocardiogram (ECG) to see how well your heart is working
* X-ray of your chest

How is it treated?

It is important to get to the hospital as soon as possible if you suspect a stroke. Many large hospitals are now treating strokes caused by blood clots with clot-dissolving medicines. These medicines can cause the symptoms to stop very quickly. They can prevent long-term disability or death. This treatment works only if the medicines are given within the first 3 to 6 hours after the stroke began.

All strokes require careful observation, especially in the first 24 hours. In addition to bed rest, you will probably need an IV and oxygen. Underlying medical problems that may have caused the stroke, such as high blood pressure or heart rhythm problems, will be treated.

Rehabilitation may start at the hospital or at a nursing facility. Most stroke rehab programs last several weeks to several months after you leave the hospital. The program consists of physical therapy, occupational therapy and, if needed, speech therapy.

* Physical therapy helps you regain muscle strength and teaches you ways to move safely with weak or paralyzed muscles.
* Occupational therapy helps you relearn ways of eating, dressing and grooming
* Speech therapy may help you, if you have problems with swallowing, speaking or understanding words

How long will the effects last?

Recovery depends on the extent of the brain injury. Some improvement may occur rapidly within the first few days and weeks after the stroke. Other improvement may occur more gradually. Rehabilitation may include physical therapy to strengthen muscles, occupational therapy to teach such things as dressing and eating, and speech therapy, if needed. If recovery does not begin within 1 to 2 weeks of the stroke, some muscle movement and speech may not return. However, some people continue to regain speech and muscle strength up to 1 year after a stroke. By the end of the rehab program, your healthcare can tell you more accurately what further recovery you can expect.

How can I prevent a stroke from occurring?

* If you have high blood pressure, it is essential that you control it with medicine.
* If you have diabetes, monitor and control your blood sugar.
* If you have an irregular or fast heart rate, you may need to take medicine such as Warfarin (coumadin), aspirin, or clopidogrel. Talk with your healthcare provider About this.
* Keep your diet low in fat to decrease the risk of developing fatty deposits in your Blood vessels
* Exercise every day according to your healthcare provider's recommendations.
* Keep a healthy weight.

The information about a stroke, that I have shared with you, is intended to inform and educate and is not a replacement for medical evaluation, advice, diagnosis or treatment by a healthcare professional.

Now on the subject of Congestive Heart Failure, in which I developed in my eight year of hemodialysis treatment. I would like to share more literature, that I have obtained from my health insurance provider. Read on.

Congestive Heart Failure:

What is heart failure?

Heart failure means your heart does not pump as well as it should. When the heart is unable to pump effectively, not enough blood reaches the organs and tissues of your body. The kidneys help the body get rid of fluid. And when the kidneys get less blood, they hold on to salt and water. This causes extra fluid to back up into the lungs causing difficulty with breathing. Fluid build up can also cause swelling of your feet, ankles, and legs. That is why the condition is called Congestive Heart Failure.

Signs and Symptoms:

*   **Swelling of the feet and/or ankles**
*   **Tire easily**
*   **Shortness of breath even when resting**

When prescribed medication and treatment plan to follow, remember these important facts:

*   Review the prescription handout on each new medication
*   Know actions, side effects and how to take prescribed medication
*   Always carry a list of your medications and keep enough for emergencies

Glo tip: Keeping a file on all medications prescribed, as well as knowing when to refill a prescribed medication, will keep you well organized and always sure of your medication and the dosage at all times.

*   Review your medication; indications, dosages, precautions, potential side Effects, interactions, an/or allergic reaction for each of the medication Prescribed.

When participating in a treatment plan, follow these steps:

Check your weight every day at the same time, with the same amount of clothing and after emptying your bladder.

If there is a weight gain of more than 2 pounds in one day or 5 or more pounds in 5 days, increase your medication dosage as ordered by your doctor.

Restrict salt intake to 2000 mg/day to help prevent fluid retention, you may also be asked to limit the fluid you drink, especially patients with chronic kidney disease.

Safety and Mobility is very important for the patient - such as:
Maintaining a daily activity plan as ordered by the doctor
Alternate exercise or activity with rest periods to avoid fatigue

Prevent Complications include:

Avoid drinking alcohol
If you smoke, please stop
Get a Flu vaccination every year
Get a Pneumovax vaccine, if not previously vaccinated

Notify your health care provider as soon as possible if you have any of the following signs of increased fluid retention:

Need to use more pillows at night to breathe
Tiring easily with your normal activity
Worsening shortness of breath at rest or with activity
Lightheadedness or dizziness while sitting
A cough that does not go away, and is intolerable
Significant side effects from medications
New or increased irregularities in heart rate
Sleeping problems, including waking up to catch your breath, sleeping in a recliner or using pillows due to labored breathing when laying flat.

CRISIS PLAN: Very Important

Call 911 or have someone take you to the nearest Emergency Room, if you have:

Severe shortness of breath and/or difficulty breathing
Coughing up pink foamy mucus
Chest pain, chest pressure, any chest discomfort not relieved by nitroglycerin
Fainting and/or loss of consciousness

What is Protein?

Protein consist of building blocks called amino acids. Your body is able to make some amino acids, but not all of them. Those which your body cannot make, must be obtained from the diet, (renal diet that is), and are called essential amino acids. There are two types of protein found in foods, and if a protein has all the essential amino acids, it is called a high biological value, or good quality protein.

High Biological Protein is found in eggs and eggs whites, fish, chicken, turkey, pork, lamb, beef, veal and tofu. Good quality proteins are used more efficiently by the body and create fewer waste products. Therefore, it is important that most of the protein in your diet come from good quality proteins.

The second type of protein is referred to as Low Biological Protein Value or Low Quality Protein, because one or more essential amino acids are missing. The body uses lower quality protein less effectively than high quality proteins. Vegetables, legumes, nuts, breads and other starches contain lower quality protein. Both high and low quality proteins will be included in your healthy diet.

NOTE: HOWEVER, SOME PROTEIN FOODS NEED TO BE LIMITED DUE TO HIGH POTASSIUM OR PHOSPHORUS CONTENT.

HOW MUCH PROTEIN IS ENOUGH?

Each time you have dialysis treatment, a little protein is lost from your body. By eating plenty of protein-enriched foods, it will replace these losses and supply your body with the protein that it needs. If you do not eat enough protein, you may feel weak, fatigue, lose muscle, and most importantly have difficulty fighting infections.

A DIALYSIS PATIENT NEEDS TO EAT SIX TO TEN OUNCES OF PROTEIN IN ORDER TO MAINTAIN CONTNUED GOOD HEALTH. (Note: a minimum of 8 ounces is preferred for peritoneal dialysis patients, because protein is removed so much more easily from the body than with hemo dialysis.

Glo's tip:

Try to include a good portion of a high protein food at every meal. Try to eat the high protein food first just in case you get full quickly. And even though, milk and cheese are very good sources of protein, it's very threatening to dialysis patients, because it contains the enemy, **PHOSPHORUS.**

NOTE: DIALYSIS PATIENTS NEED TO LIMIT THEIR INTAKE OF HIGH PHOSPHORUS FOODS
TO ONE SMALL SERVING A DAY.

For instance: a ½ cup of yogurt, ½ cup milk, and one (1) ounce of cheese

This is very important, because if you don't you'll have one of those itching saga, like I experience from time to time. I am a very serious cheese lover, I don't have trouble with milk or yogurt, because I don't particularly like either one. I still until this very day, have a problem staying away from cheese or dishes cooked with cheese. After all, I grew up on cheese, and it isn't as easy to just stop eating cheese. Don't get me wrong, I tried very hard to follow my renal diet, but when it comes to cheese, I tend to be very naughty. I feel that I'm pretty much a model patient, I've gotten in the habit of reading the ingredients on just about everything I purchase at the grocery store. If you are like me and show a great concern for the maintaining of good health on dialysis, you will pay attention to what foods you purchase and how you prepare your meals at home.

I CAN'T STRESS THIS ENOUGH, FOODS HIGH IN PROTEIN ALSO CONTAIN PHOSPHORUS, OUR ENEMY.

I know that I have shared in my first book "My Renal Life" (I know it, I live it), what albumin is all about, it bares repeating, because this part of survival with dialysis, doesn't change much, so if you don't have my first book, I am still pleased to share these important facts, that can definitely help you to manage good health with dialysis treatment.

What is Albumin?

Albumin is a protein found in your body.

Maintaining a 4.0 albumin level will help you to:

> Fight infections
> Build and repair your body tissues
> Heal wounds much better
> Keep you from becoming sick less often
> Have less hospitalization
> Keep you more energized

To maintain the albumin level, you need two to three meals and one to two snacks a day to get enough protein and calories to keep up your albumin and strength.

To attempt to get the amount of protein you need per day, this small list of foods with their ounces measured will help you to plan your meals to maintain the 4.0 albumin level you need to keep your proteins up:

> 3 ounces of a regular hamburger patty
> 4 ounces of beef steak (3"x4")
> 3 ounces of fish fillet (3"x3")
> 3 ounces of ½ chicken breast
> 3 ounces of regular pork chop
> 3 ounces of shrimp (5 medium)
> 1 ounce of one (1) whole egg
> 1 ounce of two egg whites
> And don't forget our vegetarians - 2 to 3 ounces of one (1) soy burger

NOTE: REMEMBER ALBUMIN NORMAL RANGE IS - 4.0 OR GREATER

Here is a list of some of the protein foods and the grams (amount) of protein that they contain, this list range from low to higher to highest protein foods.

To 21.0 grams - Low Protein Foods: *Note: Based on a 3 oz serving fresh and cooked, unless otherwise stated for all categories*
Beef, ground, lean - 21.0
Beef, ground, regular - 20.5
Duck, domestic, roasted - 20.5
Egg Substitute, - 11.0
Egg white, 1 large - 3.5
Egg whole, 1 large - 6.3
Veal, rib - 20.4

From 21.1 - 25.1 grams - Higher Protein Foods:
Beef, ground, extra lean - 21.6
Beef, rib, lean - 23.2
Beef, round, eye, lean - 24.6
Chicken, dark meat - 24.4
Lamb, leg, domestic, lean, cooked - 24.1
Lamb, rib, domestic, lean, cooked - 22.2
Pork, leg, fresh, lean - 25.0
Pork roast, fresh, lean, roasted - 24.4
Pork, spareribs, fresh, braised - 24.7
Turkey, dark - 24.0

25.1 or more grams - Highest Protein Foods: *Note: these foods should be limited or avoided as much as possible - keeping your proteins up, is very important to maintaining continued good health with dialysis.*
Beef, round, bottom, lean - 26.9   veal, leg - 30.7
Beef, top sirloin, lean - 25.8
Chicken, white meat - 27.6
Lamb, loin, domestic, lean, cooked - 25.5
Lamb, shoulder, domestic, lean, cooked - 30.2
Pork chops, fresh, lean, broiled - 25.7
Turkey, light - 25.1

Seafood - Another great source of protein, especially those dialysis patients that are vegetarians.

To 17.0 grams - Low Protein Seafood: (*Note: if you have protein issues, as I have had on occasion, especially since transitioning to PD, then you may have to add some more protein to your diet, because if you eat any seafood from this list, you may have to eat more than a 3 oz serving to get the recommended amount of protein that you need for that day).*
Clams, mixed species, raw - 10.9
Crab, Alaska King, cooked - 16.5
Oyster, cooked - 7.5
Oyster, raw - six (6) medium - 5.9
Scallop, cooked - 6 large - 16.8
Shrimp, six (6) large - 9.6

From 17.1 to 21 grams - Higher Protein Seafood:
Cod, cooked - 19.5
Crab, blue, cooked - 17.2
Flounder, cooked - 20.5
Haddock, cooked - 20.6
Lobster, cooked - 17.4
Ocean Perch, cooked - 20.3
Pollock, cooked - 20.0
Fillet of Sole, cooked - 20.5
Trout, Rainbow, cooked - 20.6
Tuna, white, canned in water - 20.1

21.1 or more grams - Highest Protein Seafood:
Halibut, cooked - 22.7
Salmon - 23.2
Swordfish, cooked - 21.6
Tuna salad, 1 cup - 32.9
Tuna light, canned in oil - 24.8
Tuna, yellowfin, cooked - 25.5

Dairy - Low, High, Highest of protein foods: *Note: Be very careful with these foods or products, because it will effect your phosphorus levels, if you were to over indulge. The grams are as stated.*

From 7.9 grams - Low Protein Dairy Food:
Buttermilk, ½ cup - 4.1
Cheese, blue - 1 oz - 6.0
Cheese, cheddar - 1 oz - 7.0
Cheese, cream - 1 tbsp - 1.1
Cheese, cream, fat free - 1 tbsp - 2.3
Cheese, feta - 1 oz - 4.0
Cheese, mozzarella - 7.8
Cheese, parmesan cheese - 1 tbsp - 2.1
Cheese, provolone - 1 oz - 7.3
Ice cream, vanilla - ½ cup - 2.3
Ice cream, vanilla, light (50%) - ½ cup - 2.5
Sherbert, orange - 1 cup - 1.6
Yogurt, frozen, vanilla - ½ cup - 2.9
Yogurt, plain, whole - 1 cup - 7.9

From 8 to 12 grams - Higher Protein Dairy Food:
Cheese, swiss - 1 oz - 8.1
Milk, 1% - 1 cup - 8.0
Milk, 2% - 1 cup - 8.1
Milk, evaporated, nonfat - ½ cup - 9.7
Milk, non-fat - 1 cup - 8.4
Milk, whole - 1 cup - 8.0
Yogurt, plain, low fat - 1 cup - 11.9

12.1 or more grams - Highest Protein Dairy Food:
Cheese, cottage, creamed - 1 cup - 26.0
Cheese, cottage, low fat (2% milk fat) - 1 cup - 31.0
Cheese, cottage, non-fat - 1 cup - 25.0
Cheese, ricotta, part skim milk - 1 cup - 28.0
Cheese, ricotta, whole milk - 1 cup - 27.7
Milk, condensed, sweetened - ½ cup - 12.1
Milk, dry, nonfat instant - ½ cup - 12.2
Yogurt, plain, skim - 1 cup - 13.0

Legumes and Nuts - Low, High, Highest of Protein: *Note: All legumes (dried beans and peas) are high in potassium and phosphorus, and also poor quality protein, which can cause an elevated BUN (Urea Nitrogen) level.*

To 7.9 grams - Low Protein - based on a ½ cup serving or as stated:
Beans, black, boiled - 7.6
Beans, kidney, boiled - 7.7
Beans, lima - 7.3
Beans, navy, boiled - 7.9
Beans, pinto - 7.0
Beans, refried - 6.9
Chickpeas, boiled - 7.3
Cowpeas, cooked from raw, drained - 2.6
Pecans - 2 oz - 5.2
Soymilk - 3.8

From 8 to 12 grams - Higher Protein - based on a ½ cup serving or as stated:
Beans, white - 9.5
Cashew, dry, roasted - 2 oz - 8.7
Cashew, oil, roasted - 2 oz - 9.2
Chestnuts, European - 2 oz - 9.1
Hazelnuts - 2 oz - 8.5
Peanut Butter - 2 tbsp - 8.0
Peas, split - 8.2
Soy hamburger patty - 2.5 oz - 12.0
Tofu, silken, raw - 4 oz - 9.6
Tofu, soft, raw - 4 oz - 9.0
Walnuts, English - 2 oz - 8.6

12.1 or more grams - Highest Protein - based on a ½ cup serving or as stated:
Almonds - 2 oz - 12.1   Tofu, firm, raw - 4 oz - 13.0
Beans, soy, cooked - 14.3   Soy chicken patty - 2.5 oz - 13.0
Lentils, cooked - 17.9   Pistachios, dry, roasted - 2 oz - 12.1
Peanuts, dry, roasted - 2 oz - 13.4
Peanuts, oil, roasted - 2 oz - 14.9
Pine nuts, dried - 2 oz - 13.6

Grains and Cereals - based on a 1 cup serving or 1 slice, unless otherwise stated:

To 2.9 grams - Low Protein
Bread, French - ½" slice - 2.2
Bread, Italian - 1.8
Bread, Oatmeal - 2.3
Bread, Wheat - 2.7
Cereal, crispy rice - 2.1
Cereal, corn flakes - 1.8
Cereal, corn squares - 2.2
Cereal, rice squares - 1.9
Doughnut, plain - 2.4
Rolls, dinner (brown and served) - 1 roll - 2.4

From 3 to 6 grams - Higher Protein
Biscuits, plain - 2 ½" - 4.2
Bread, pita, white - 6 ½" - 5.5
Cereal, cream of wheat, regular - 3.8
Croissants, butter, 1 croissant - 4.7
Croutons, seasoned - 4.3
English Muffin - 1 whole - 4.4
Muffin, blueberry, pre-made - 1 muffin - 3.1
Oatmeal, plain instant - 1 packet - 4.4
Rice, brown, cooked - 5.0
Rice, white, cooked - 4.3
Rolls, hot dog or hamburger - 1 roll - 3.7
Rolls, Kaiser - 1 roll - 5.6

6.1 or more grams - Highest Protein
Bagel, eggs - 3 ½" - 7.5
Bread crumbs, seasoned - 17.0
Bread stuffing, from mix - 6.4
Couscous, dry - 22.1
Macaroni, cooked - 6.7
Noodles, egg, cooked - 7.6
Rice, wild, cooked - 6.5
Spaghetti, cooked - 6.7
Wheat flour, white - 12.9
Wheat flour, whole grain - 16.44

What is Phosphorus?

Phosphorus is a mineral that works together with calcium to keep your bones strong and healthy. People with kidney disease have to be careful with their diet, because their kidneys won't get rid of this extra phosphorus.

Phosphorus and Calcium should be in balance in your body. When the phosphorus in your blood becomes too high, you disturb the balance of the phosphorus and calcium. Your body will sense this imbalance and the parathyroid gland in your neck will send a message to take calcium from your bones, which results into Renal Bone Disease. *Dialysis will not correct high levels of phosphorus), so that's where you (the patient) comes in, you need to watch your intake of phosphorus, by learning the low, moderate, and high content of phosphorus in foods. In instances when the phosphorus becomes too high in your blood, you may experience uncontrollable itching, that may require an anti-itching medication for relief. However the medication will not remove phosphorus from your body. You still have to do your part in watching your phosphorus intake.*

YOU CAN CONTROL THE PHOSPHORUS IN YOUR BODY, BY LIMITING THE PHOSPHORUS IN YOUR DIET, AND ALSO I CAN"T STRESS THIS ENOUGH - PLEASE DON'T FORGET TO TAKE YOUR PHOSPHORUS BINDERS, IT WILL MAKE LIFE SO MUCH EASIER, AND IS VERY BENEFICIAL TO MAINTAINING GOOD HEALTH.

The purpose of the binders, is to grab or bound the phosphorus in your food, before it can reach your blood-stream.

Just remember that if you continue to eat high phosphorus foods and neglect to take your binders, *LOOK-OUT! - you'll start having uncontrollable itching, your bones will get brittle, you'll get hardening of the blood vessels and body organs which leads to heart attack, and the potential for bone disease and calcification in soft tissues, (such as: the heart and lungs), pain in the bones and joints, and red eyes. I saw a display in the PD patients department, and if you saw what I saw, , you wouldn't want your phosphorus to get that out of control ever, which may result in the development of calcifications in your eyes, foot, etc. etc., it looks so creepy and hideous.* Take it from me, try hard, I mean real hard to keep your phosphorus levels in range, preferably under 5.5 O.K? I learned this the hard way, I sure wish someone would've imbedded this in my head, maybe if I had knowledge of this on my initial start of hemo dialysis treatment, it would have saved me from some of those uncontrollable itching attacks I've had in the pass, causing damage to my skin. It's an ongoing battle for me to stay away from cheese.

I've learned even though your binders maybe prescribed a certain way, you don't ever continue to eat the same, you may have to take extras. Even if you eat a fresh fruit take some binders. Any snack you consume take those binders PLEASE. When you dine out, please don't forget to take your binders with you. Honey, I have a two story house, and I keep binders downstairs in the kitchen, as well as upstairs in my bedroom and craft room where I spend a lot of my time. I also keep binders in a compartment of my key chain for emergencies. So you know I religiously keep binders with me at all times.

Sharing my experience moment: I refer to this list on the regular for many years during my dialysis journey, and it has helped me to have a better understanding of the importance of paying close attention to the nutritional facts, that has also helped me to prepare renal friendly meals, that can accommodate my family as well. And as I know, that this renal diet ain't no joke, it can be very complex, and a lot of drama to abide by, but with faith and determination, yes, it can be done. Getting into the habit of reading the labels, when you go grocery shopping, will also help in managing your health with a renal diet. It is mandatory that the nutritional facts are displayed on products these days, but as far as how much phosphorus is in its contents, you can only see that the product has some form of phosphorus in the ingredients, but not how much. You can always check this list that I share with you, about how much phosphorus some of these products contain. Here is a list of some of the common forms of phosphorus..

Common Hidden Sources of Phosphorus: (Most foods when you read the label, you can find out if it contains some source of phosphorus, but it may not tell you how much phosphorus it contains, so use your own judgement when eating a food that contains phosphorus and please take your binders.

Phosphoric Acid
Pyrophosphates
Hexametaphosphate
Dicalcium Phosphate
Monocalcium Phosphate
Sodium Phosphate

What is Calcium?

Calcium is a mineral that works together with phosphorus to keep your bones strong and healthy. Milk and other dairy foods are naturally high in calcium. Some non-dairy foods may have calcium added. Avoid calcium fortified foods.

When grocery shopping, try to avoid buying foods with the following calcium labels:

- Good Source of Calcium
- Calcium Fortified
- Excellent Source of Calcium
- Calcium Enriched

Snack Crackers, Granola Bar, Breakfast Cereals, Pancake/Muffin Mixes, Frozen Waffles, Juices, Margarines & Powdered Drink Mixes - Check label for added Calcium. All in all, just get in the habit of buying foods that have no added calcium.

AND REMEMBER TOO MUCH CALCIUM CAN WEAKEN YOUR BONES ALSO, JUST LIKE PHOSPHORUS CAN.

NOTE: NORMAL RANGE FOR CALCIUM - 8.4 - 9.4

What is Calcium & Phosphorus Corrected?

Calcium & Phosphorus = Product - Normal product is important for healthy bones and heart. Keeping your phosphorus levels low and taking your binders as prescribed, can help in maintaining a good calcium and phosphorus product.

I know all this sounds quite complicated, so let me break it down to you, your calcium, phosphorus and PTH all work together hand in hand. What it all boils down to is keeping that muscle happy - (meaning your heart).

CALCIUM & PHOSPHORUS PRODUCT - NORMAL RANGE - Less than 55

What is PTH?

PTH - is the Parathyroid Hormone. This also helps to keep your bones healthy, when it is in normal range. When the phosphorus in your blood becomes too high, you disturb the balance of the phosphorus and calcium. Your body will sense this imbalance and the parathyroid gland in your neck will send a message to take calcium from your bones. This eventually makes the bones become brittle, because apparently too much calcium has been removed from your bones. And the result of this is, renal bone disease, and *calcification in soft tissues, such as the heart and lungs.*
Elevated levels increase your risk for renal bone disease.

PTH INTACT - (PARATHYROID HORMONE) - NORMAL RANGE - 150 TO 300

My Story: I wasn't having any problems with my PTH level during my ten year run with hemo dialysis treatment, but a few months after beginning peritoneal dialysis treatment, I began to have issues with my PTH level rising, and rapidly approaching the 1,000 level mark. During this time, my previous neprologist constantly made changes to my vitamin D, which was rocatrol, I started out taking two pills twice a day, and then it was changed to every other day, and not on the weekend, and I went through this for almost four months, until I was assigned to a new neprologist, who reviewed my records, and immediately was concerned about my PTH levels being so elevated, he couldn't understand why I didn't have some of my thyroid glands removed, so he immediately scheduled the surgery to have my glands removed. I had the surgical procedure done to remove parathyroid glands in my neck, so this can eliminate robbing calcium from my bones, and that I may not ever develop renal bone disease. The only reason why this may happens, is because when you are in end stage renal failure, the kidneys can no longer balance your phosphorus and calcium in your body. After having the surgical procedure, I wasn't allowed to be discharged that day, I was then admitted, and was told by my doctor, that I needed to be monitored, because with this procedure it is common to have a plummeted calcium level. And yes, that is what happened, but the nurse monitored me very closely through the night, blood was drawn several times during the night, and when it indicated that the calcium had decreased, (and trust me, you will have a side effect, that indicates that the calcium has dropped, I experienced tingling in my fingers, and when I tried to grab at something, it was truly difficult, it was almost like I was learning for the first time, how to reach for something. That is why it is so important to keep your phosphorus in normal range. I know that it is important to keep the sodium, potassium, phosphorus and protein in normal range, but as you can see from my own experience, the calcium is very important to keep in normal range also. Since the thyroid gland removal, I've been taking levothyroxine for over ten years now on a daily basis, and of course sensipar, to help the calcium stay in balance.

Cholesterol

Cholesterol - To keep your levels normal in your body, try eating foods that are low in cholesterol and fat, if that doesn't work for you, you may be prescribed a medication to lower your cholesterol in your body.

For the last five years I've had an issue with cholesterol. And the prescription medicine that I take, I had to eliminate liver (in which I love) from my renal diet.

CHOLESTEROL NORMAL RANGE - 100 TO 200

Note: Avocados contain no cholesterol. Their fat and fiber can help lower blood cholesterol.
But also remember, dialysis patients if you have to watch your potassium intake, then don't indulge in too much avocados.

Glo's Tip: Use mashed avocados on bread in place of mayonnaise more often, it also gives your sandwich a great taste.

Use tub margarine to limit the cholesterol in your diet
Use olive oil and canola oil in your cooking

Triglycerides - Triglycerides are fats normally found in your blood.

TRIGLYCERIDES NORMAL RANGE - BELOW 200

Facts about fats in foods:

Note: Frying add fats to foods
For Example: The vegetable - potato
The greater the surface area of potato exposed to fat or oil, the higher the fat content
Roast potato - (3 oz.) - 5g fat, 65 calories
Fries - (large, 3 oz.) - 12g fat, 220 calories
Fries - (small, 3 oz.) - 15g fat, 265 calories
Potato Chips - (3 oz.) - 30g fat, 450 calorie

Healthy Fats

Fats in food provide energy, which help the body absorb certain vitamins. Fats from seafood and the oils from vegetables, nuts, and seeds provide health benefits that can protect your blood vessels and reduce your risk of developing type 2 diabetes and heart disease. These are called unsaturated fats, which are usually liquid at room temperature.

Super healthy fats to cook with: (olive oil, canola, and peanut oil). They lower harmful LDL cholesterol in the blood, which raise helpful HDL cholesterol and cut Triglycerides, which eases the risk for type 2 diabetes disease and heart disease.

Polyunsaturated Fats:

Corn, sunflower, safflower, flaxseed, soybean, and fatty fish (such as albacore tuna and salmon), these fats are rich in omega-3 and omega-6 fatty acids. These fats lower cholesterol, But Note: In some cases they may also lower helpful HDL cholesterol.

Unhealthy Fats

Saturated Fats:

There are some types of fats that can be harmful to your health, which can increase your chances of developing type 2 diabetes, heart disease, blood vessel problems, and stroke. The most damaging fats are saturated fats and trans fats, which are usually solid or semisolid at room temperature. Of course it is impossible to avoid all harmful fats, because they are contained in many foods, so be wise, and try to cut back on fats in your foods.

Fat that can raise your LDL cholesterol - full-fat dairy products, butter, coconut oil, palm oil, and poultry skin. This can put you at risk for heart disease and diabetes complications.

Trans Fats:

Vegetable oils, margarines, shortening, some processed and fast foods can raise harmful LDL and total cholesterol.

What is Carbohydrates?

Carbohydrates are the sugars, starches and fiber that come from fruits, vegetables and whole grains.

Note: For individuals who are at risk of Type 2 Diabetes and those who have it, whole grains and fiber are especially beneficial because they do not increase blood sugar and insulin as much as white bread and white rice.

Healthy Carbohydrates:

Whole grains - the seeds of grasses such as wheat, oats, rice, corn, rye, barley, millet, kasha, and quinoa - are linked to a lower risk of Type 2 Diabetes, heart disease, and stroke. They are rich in vitamin B, calcium, magnesium and phosphorus - which in dialysis patient - too much phosphorus can be harmful,

Unhealthy Carbohydrates:

Note: White bread, white rice and white pasta - are digested faster than whole grains and can quickly raise the blood glucose. When the outer husk is stripped from these grains, these processed, refined grains lose most of their nutrients and fiber.

Fiber:

Fiber found mainly in whole grains such as wheat, oats, and rye is very beneficial for people who have type 2 diabetes or the individual who wants to avoid type 2 diabetes. Fiber reduces blood sugar and the need for insulin and improves blood cholesterol also.

Note: Fiber is the indigestible part of plant foods.

What is Iron Saturation?

Iron Saturation is the amount of iron available in your blood. Iron is needed to build red blood cells and to prevent anemia.

IRON SATURATION NEEDS TO BE 20 - 50% IN YOUR BODY

What is Ferritin?

Ferritin is your iron stores. (meaning the amount of iron stored in your body)

FERRITIN NORMAL RANGE - 100 TO 800

What is Iron?

Iron is a very important mineral that is needed for many body functions. Iron is needed to make the red blood cells that carry oxygen through the entire body. Low iron levels are referred to as "iron deficiency".

Common causes of low iron levels in dialysis patients are:

- Blood loss from blood tests or dialysis treatments
- Poor absorption of iron from food
- Not eating enough high-iron foods

Without enough iron you may develop the following:

- Low energy level and difficulty concentrating
- Pale skin color and thin curved nails
- Anemia (a low hematocrit and a low hemoglobin level)

When you have blood test done monthly at the unit, you can find out if your iron levels are low- the Iron Saturation and Ferritin will tell how much iron is available in your blood, and how much iron you have stored in your body.

If your iron levels are low, intravenous (IV) iron may be administered during hemo dialysis treatment, or your doctor may prescribe iron pills, or both, also along with epogen shots (EPO), but for peritoneal dialysis patients EPO shot of course, and in some cases iron pills are also prescribed.

If you are taking iron pills:

- Take it separate from your phosphate binders
- Take it between meals or at bedtime
- On hemo dialysis days, take your iron after treatment

- Do not take it with dairy products, coffee, tea, or alcohol
- Take the amount of iron supplement the doctor prescribes for you (there are instances where the dosage could be changed or stop)
- Increase your intake of high iron foods such as: lean meat, iron-fortified cereals Enriched rice
- Use an iron skillet for cooking (if one is available)

(EDUCATION FOR YOUR INFORMATION) - Iron is found in foods from both plants and animals, however: Iron from animal food sources is better used by the body, vitamin C and protein foods help absorb iron from plant foods, Strawberries, tangerines and enriched cranberry juice are renal-friendly sources of Vitamin C (limit to ½ cup servings).

Glo's Tip: Read food labels and look for 20% or more iron per serving

What is Sodium?

Sodium is an important mineral also that the body needs in very small amounts. Its major functions are to regulate your blood pressure and to maintain the proper amount of fluid in your blood and body cells.

In healthy kidneys, excess sodium that is eaten is eliminated through the urine. But when kidney function decreases, the excess sodium may cause fluid to stay in your body. This may result in swelling and high blood pressure. Foods high in sodium will also increase your thirst, causing you to drink more fluid than you should. Most dialysis patients should have about **2,000 milligrams** each day of sodium, that's half the amount that most people eat.

Try to avoid the salt-shaker, it's a big step in reducing sodium intake. Processed foods usually have sodium added as a part of the processing and preparation making them very high in sodium. *WHAT OUT!*

NOTE: SODIUM NORMAL RANGE - 135 - 148

Listed below are salty foods that a dialysis patient should avoid as much as possible:

Salted, smoked and cured meats such as:

(Glo's comment: come now, one hot dog isn't going to kill you, just know your limits)

Ham	Hot Dogs
Luncheon Meats	Salt Pork
Corned Beef	Smoked Salmon
Beef & Pork Bacon	

(Glo's Tip: Even though it is suggested that you don't eat bacon, it's ok to have a strip with your eggs and grits for breakfast, just don't over indulge or make a habit of it, every once and awhile is o.k.)

Canned, boxed or packaged prepared foods such as:

Soups	Instant Potatoes
Gravies	Bisquick Macaroni and Cheese
Spaghetti sauce	Waffle Mix
Hamburger Helper	Seasoning Mixes
Beef Stew	Vegetable Juice
Boxed Macaroni and Cheese	Salad Dressing - (Store Bought)

(Glo's Tip: It would help if you would make your own salad dressing, so that way you can control the intake of sodium, potassium, and phosphorus it will contain)

Note: Check out the section - Salad Dressing - for some of my homemade recipes for salad dressing

Frozen prepared entrees and dinners
Food cured in brine such as: Olives, Pickles, Sauerkraut, and Relish

Salted Snack Foods, Salt, Sea Salt, MSG and seasoning salts such as: Garlic, and Onion Salt, catsup, mustard, worchestire sauce, soy sauce and horseradish: (Most of my recipes are prepared with worchestire sauce, but I only use a small portion - ½ tsp for flavor. Because the nutritional facts are mandatory on products these days, you should get in the habit of reading the labels when you go grocery shopping. It can help you to find hidden sources of sodium.

(Glo's Tip: You can really control the amount of sodium in your diet by cooking most of your meals from scratch. Try experimenting with different seasonings and discover fresh new taste to your liking. Bring out natural flavors by using lemon juice, vinegars, herbs and spices-(Mrs. Dash makes a variety of herbal seasonings). My favorites are: Mrs. Dash table blend, and garlic and herb).

Below is a list of some herbs, spices and flavorings that you can try, to enhance the flavor in your cooking:

Allspice

Almond extract

Anise

Basil

Bay Leaf

Caraway seed

Mint

Mustard, dry or seed

Nutmeg

Onion, fresh juice or powder juice

Orange extract

Paprika

Cardamom

Celery seed

Chili powder

Chives

Cinnamon

Cilantro

Cloves

Cumin

Curry

Dill Fennel

Garlic, fresh, juice or powder

Ginger

Horseradish root

Horseradish root w/no salt

Juniper

Lemon juice

Lemon juice extract

Mace

Marjoram

Rice Wine Vinegar

Variety of Flavored Wine Vinegars

Pepper, fresh - bell pepper (green, red, orange, or yellow)

Pepper, black, red, or white

Peppermint extract

Pimento peppers for garnish

Poppy seeds

Parsley (fresh or flakes)

Purslane

Rosemary

Saffron

Sage

Savory

Sesame seeds

Sorrel

Sugar

Tarragon

Thyme

Turmeric

Vanilla extract

Maple extract

Wine

When grocery shopping, some products may have these definitions labeled (with salt contents) as follows:

Sodium free - mean less than 5 mg of sodium per serving
Very low sodium - mean only 35 mg of sodium per serving
Low sodium - less than 140 mg of sodium per serving
Reduced sodium - usual level of sodium is reduced by 25%
Light or lite in sodium - usual level of sodium is reduced by 50%

Common hidden sources of salt: (Hint: if sodium is in the word - Sodium = Salt)

Sodium ascorbate
Sodium benzoate
Sodium biphosphate
Sodium casein ate

Monosodium glutamate (MSG)
Sodium nitrite or nitrate
Disodium phosphate
Sodium gluconate

The Importance Of Fluid Restriction

Fluid is a very important factor when it comes to having adequate dialysis treatment.

Dry Weight - is the weight at which your body has no excess fluid and your blood pressure is well controlled.

Fluid Weight - is the weight you gain between dialysis treatments from the fluids you consume.

The fluids consumed between dialysis sessions will build up in the blood and tissues, causing swelling in your ankles and feet. Fluid can also collect in the lungs or around your heart causing shortness of breath or congestive heart failures. Fluid gained between treatments is removed during dialysis. Fluid does not show in swelling or breathing problems for some people, but they have problems getting fluid removed to reach the dry weight during dialysis. If you drink too much fluid it becomes more difficult to remove in one dialysis session. As a result excess fluid gains can cause low blood pressure, cramps, nausea and vomiting toward the end of dialysis treatment.

Between dialysis treatments, your fluid weight gain should be about 1 to 3 kilograms or 2 to 6 pounds.

FOR YOUR INFORMATION: TWO (2) CUPS OF FLUID WEIGHT ½ KILOGRAM OR 1 POUND.

Note: However your total fluid intake per day will vary according to your kidney function.

Below is a chart on common measurements:

Common Measurements

| 1 tablespoon | = ½ ounce | = 15cc |
| 2 tablespoon | = 1 ounce | = 30cc |

½ cup	= 4 ounces	= 120cc
1 cup	= 8 ounces	= 240cc
1 ½ cup	= 12 ounces (soda can)	= 360cc
2 cups	= 16 ounces	= 500cc
4 cups	= 32 ounces (1 quart)	= 1,000cc

FOR YOUR INFORMATION: FOODS THAT ARE LIQUID AT ROOM TEMPERATURE WILL CONTRIBUTE TO YOUR FLUID GAIN.

Below is a chart of common sources of fluid:

Water	Ice
Juice	Tea
Coffee	Soda
Milk	Ice Cream
Sherbet	Soup
Gelatin	Popsicles
Syrups in canned fruit	

In the beginning, if you have difficulty controlling your fluid intake, try these tips:

If you get thirsty, try sucking on frozen grapes, ice chips, chilled lemon.

(Glo's Tip: an 12oz. Glass of crushed ice, will melt to half a glass of water). It's better than drinking a glass of water, you will cut down tremendously on your fluid intake.

What is Glucose?

Glucose is blood sugar. If you have diabetes, it is very important that you keep your blood sugar at the normal fasting range at the beginning of the day, and below 160 about two (2) hours after meals.

In some cases when the glucose is too low. It maybe from not eating enough food or skipping meals, and this can cause low blood sugar levels.

GLUCOSE NORMAL FASTING RANGE - 80 TO 160

Using a sugar substitutes:

The good thing is artificial sweeteners are carb-free. Instead of using sugar, a calorie-free sugar alternative should be used in cooking. They can help you lose weight or maintain a healthy weight. Sugar rich foods tend to be high in calories and low in nutrients-and most importantly, they raise blood glucose. However a non-sugar sweetener has no effect on blood glucose.

The most popular sugar substitutes are sucralose, aspartame, and saccharin. The sweetener sucralose doesn't change when heated and is the best sweetener to use in cooking.

Note: When baking with sucralose, you may have to make adjustments, such as increasing the amount of flour in your recipe.

Using a sugar substitute doesn't necessary mean you have the luxury of overindulging. There are often lots of calories in some of the other ingredients used in your particular recipe, so it's very important to limit your portion size.

Blood Pressure- (The Highs And Lows)

WHAT ABOUT THE BLOOD PRESSURE?

The blood pressure and dialysis go hand in hand, and the blood pressure plays an important part in maintaining good health, especially when it pertains to dialysis.

Why is it important to measure your blood pressure?

Because an individuals blood pressure measurement can reflect the condition of a person's health, and high blood pressure can potentially be linked to very serious illness such as heart disease, a stroke, and kidney failure.

And even if you aren't a dialysis patient, you need to from time to time check or have your blood pressure check, because like I mentioned, your blood pressure can reflect the condition of your health and high blood pressure not controlled by an individual, can result to more serious health problems.

Some patients are walking around as we speak with hypertension (high blood pressure), and aren't really aware, and why do you think that it's called the silent killer?, (no warning, no symptoms). Most people that are hypertensive don't realize they are at risk until their health is seriously threatened.

The Standard Blood Pressure Classification

Hypertension (high blood pressure) - reading - upper number indicates - systolic - over 160

Example: 175/101

"   " - reading - bottom number indicates - diastolic - over 95

Hypotonia - (border value) - reading - systolic - 140-159, diastolic - 90-94

Hypotension - (low blood pressure) - reading - upper number indicates - systolic - under 139

Example: 119/69

- reading - bottom number indicates - diastolic - under 89

Living with the Silent Killer -
(better known as high blood pressure) -
My Story

Fact: Did you know that hypertension is one of the most common causes of chronic kidney disease, other than the diabetes disease. And did you know that 70% of the people in the United States with kidney disease have high blood pressure or diabetes or both.

My introduction with the silent killer began when I was in my mid twenties. I had just landed my first serious job, and the requirement was a complete physical, which was done by the company's employee physician. My blood pressure was taken and repeated, and it was discovered that I had hypertension (high blood pressure), and after the physical exam was over. Because of my young age, the doctor was concerned about my elevated blood pressure reading and I was referred to another doctor. It was soon apparent that I had inherited the poly cystic kidney disease from my father. I know there was a possibility that I would inherit the disease, but I was hoping that I could prevent myself from ever having to undergo hemo dialysis treatment. A blood pressure medication was immediately prescribed for me, and he also strongly suggested that I lower my sodium intake (meaning salt) in my diet. I began to take the medication prescribed and restricted my sodium intake in my diet. It didn't take very long before my blood pressure was regulated with these changes, but about a decade later, I became pregnant and my poly cystic kidney disease and hypertension labeled me as a having a high risk pregnancy and my blood pressure was carefully monitored. I didn't get very far into my pregnancy, because I developed pre clampsia at a little under six months of pregnancy and had to deliver prematurely so that the doctor could save me, in other words, my baby had a better chance of surviving than I did.

After the pregnancy, about five years later and during the start of dialysis, I was prescribed a much stronger blood pressure controlling medication, and as the years went on, my blood pressure became an issue after transplantation, and after the removal of the transplanted kidney. There was times when I was on four blood pressure controlling medications and a patch. At times I would have to seek medical attention, because my blood pressure was so out of control. It was necessary once that I was hospitalized and had strong intravenous medications to get the blood pressure under control. From this day I still have an ongoing battle with high blood pressure and also believe it or not low blood pressure from time to time.

I had an incidence where my blood pressure just kept dropping, and at the time I was prescribed a new medication to prevent myself from having a recurring stroke, but I read that this medication cause low blood pressure, but I couldn't stop the medication, because it was important that I keep taking this particular medicine.

Since becoming a peritoneal dialysis patient, my solution was changed to a weak dosage for treatment, to help me retain some fluid, so that my blood pressure will began to rise again, isn't that something. When I was on hemo dialysis, I was told to restrict my fluids, so as to not develop high blood pressure. I would eat high sodium soups or broth, to help bring my blood pressure. I then began to have a normal blood pressure again, and of course, I had to restart my blood pressure controlling medicine. I never stop taking one of the blood pressure controlling medicines, because if I would have stopped cold turkey, this would cause my pulse to rise, and that could be potentially dangerous. All in all, you learn a great deal about your medications once you become familiar with them. My husband and I take an abundance of medication between the two of us, and I have advised a system to become more familiar and more comfortable with our medication regiment. I decided that the label on the bottles wasn't enough for me to better understand my medicine, so I began to label our bottles on the top, so they cold be more easily accessible and we could get use to the dose, that we needed to take of our medicine. Also my husband and I have very good organization with our medicine, because we keep them all lined up together in one of my daughter's old easter baskets and also a plastic container of some kind.

Dialysis & Fitness

Let's not forget exercising, it can help a Dialysis Patient:

- Lose Weight
- Get better sleep
- Have better muscle tone
- Improve their blood pressure

- Lower their Cholesterol and Triglycerides
- Feel more energetic
- Improve their blood pressure
- Have good mobility

The exercise really doesn't have to be strenuous, just walking up and down the stairs, taking a brisk afternoon walk, (preferably after the sun has gone down), doing the laundry, and working in the garden, just to name a few.

Glo's Tip: I found out the hard way taking a walk when the sun was up. One day I did just that, and it was one of those very hot days. I began to sweat, and my blood pressure dropped, and that's not a good thing, because I began to feel fatigue, as though I was going to faint. So try to go out for your brisk walk, when the sun is down. O.K?

Rules for Diabetics - When it comes to Exercising?

Dialysis Patients with Diabetes, you may need to plan meals and snacks when you start an exercise program.
A drop in blood sugar may occur up to 6-10 hrs. after exercise. To avoid this happening, monitor your blood sugar both before and after exercise

But check with your doctor before starting an exercise program, OK?

The Importance of Medication

Medicines can treat and cure many health problems. However, they must be taken properly to ensure that they are safe and effective. Many medicines have powerful ingredients that interact with the human body in different ways, and diet as well as your lifestyle can sometimes have a significant impact on a drug's ability to work in the body. Certain foods, beverages, alcohol, caffeine, and even cigarettes can interact with medicines. This may make them less effective or may cause dangerous side effects or other health problems.

When you take medicine, be sure to follow your doctor's instructions carefully to obtain the maximum benefit with the least risk. Changes in a medicine's effect due to an interaction with food, alcohol or caffeine can be significant; however, there are many individual factors that influence the potential for such variations, like dose, age, weight, sex, and overall health.

What to Know
When Taking Medication

- Take your medication in a well-lit area

- Double check the label instructions to make sure you are taking the right medication and the prescribed amount at the right time.

- Follow your physician's, pharmacist's, and prescription label instructions exactly. Do not stop taking the medication without your physician's approval.

- If you forget to take a dose or several doses, don't take two or more doses together. Instead, ask your doctor or pharmacist for directions.

- If oral medications bother your stomach, try taking them with bread, crackers, or other food.

- Alcohol and some foods can change the way medications work—check the label and ask your pharmacist or doctor.

- DO NOT take "over the counter" (OTC) medications without first checking with your pharmacist or doctor. Sometimes another medication can change the way other medications work.

- DO NOT take a medication that doesn't look right or is out-dated.

- DO NOT save unused or out-dated medication to use it at another time.

- DO NOT give medication prescribed for you to other people - it could potentially hurt them.

Rules on Storing Your Medication:

- Keep your medication in its original container or in a properly labeled prescription bottle or box.

- Store your medication in a cool, dry place unless instructed otherwise by your doctor or pharmacist.

  DO NOT keep your medication in the bathroom medicine chest or cupboards; the heat and humidity may cause it to lose its effectiveness.

- Throw out any medications that has expired, has no label, or was prescribed for a particular illness that is now over.

- If you have any children or children visit your home, make sure your medications have childproof caps, and are always kept beyond the reach of children in a secured location.

Glo' Tip: Monitor closely to see if your medication has desired effects and/ or causing a problem, because take it from me, medications can cause unintended effects such as side effects, allergies, and interactions
With other medications you can be taking or in some cases some of the foods you may consume. Don't assume any symptoms is a normal side effect that you have to cope with. By all means, please call your doctor or pharmacist anytime you suspect your medications are making you sick or you notice these possible side-effects listed below: There are a number of side effects that could possibility occur.

Possible side effects, that could occur with taking medication:

Sudden fever or chills

Chest tightness, wheezing,

Rashes, (new itchiness)

Flushing of the skin

Dizziness, light-headedness, or fainting

Nausea, indigestion,

Difficulty breathing

Shortness of breath

Sweating

Bruising or bleeding

abdominal cramping

Vomiting 2-3 times or more in an hour
Constipation   Diarrhea
Difficulty urinating or starting a stream
Incontinence (difficulty controlling urine or BM)
Confusion, forgetfulness, depression, disorientation, or drowsiness
Difficulty sleeping, irritability, nervousness, restlessness, agitation
Heart palpitations
Changes in pulse or blood pressure
Dry mouth

Dialysis patients in the beginning will be prescribed a blood pressure controller, phosphorus binder, iron supplement, renal vitamins, and in some cases cholesterol controlling medication.

My Story: I started out with a four medicine regiment, and as the years went on, other medications were peritoneal dialysis, I began to have issues with my cholesterol levels rising, and I was then prescribed a cholesterol controlling medication. Also if you read the chapter on PTH, you know I had a bout with my parathyroid glands giving me static. And of course, when I have a problem with itching, I do have a medication prescribed for me. Dialysis patients from time to time have an issue with nausea and constipation, so a medication is prescribed or an over the counter medication is recommended. After developing a second minor stroke I was prescribed a medication to take daily to help in avoiding future strokes. And don't forget diarrhea comes into play from time to time also for one health issue or another, I had to eventually find a system to take my medication on time, and never forget to take them.

I take a multitude of medication, so I began to label the top of my bottles to make it more easier to learn my medicines and their dosages. Also I would prepare my medication for the week, and therefore this help me to memorized every medication I take and to keep tabs on refills. I started a folder a few years after starting dialysis, so that I can keep track of my many medication purchases and where I can purchase them. I would keep all receipts and literature given to me by the pharmacist about the medicine, why I'm taking a particular medication and the side affect that could develop. With the pharmacy plans that most patients are on, you have to learn all about your plan or plans and what medication you can afford and if there is a generic brand available. Believe me this has become high maintenance for most dialysis patients like myself. Because there are some plans that don't allow you to purchase certain medicine at certain times of the month. You see I have that situation from time to time, for instance, my medicine from time to time has to be limited or maybe taking every other day, in some cases more needs to be taken. Sometimes I have to take so little of it, that sometimes that dosage is not available, I'll have to cut the pills, so measuring is very important. Most of the time I don't stop a medication cold turkey, because sometimes that could potentially be harmful to do. I can't stress this enough, you must pay close attention to your medication regiment, and all the changes that have to be made. Keep a journal to jot down important notes and changes to your medication, when it was started, and why you were prescribed this particular medication, and most importantly keep the current dosage recorded. If you have good organization, maintaining this should become very easy for you.

My Personal Issues
With
Medication

I remember the first time I was prescribed medication, you may have read in a previous chapter in this book, when I shared the story of when I landed my first serious job, after graduating from college, the requirement was a full physical, and in completion of the physical exam, my blood pressure reading was in question, especially at my young age, after being referred to and exam by a specialist, I was prescribed a blood pressure controlling medication, and after giving birth to my premature daughter, five years later, I developed end stage renal disease, and had to start hemo dialysis treatment in a matter of months, having dialysis, I was prescribed a much stronger blood pressure controlling medication, phosphorus binders, iron, and vitamins (such as folic acid and renal vitamins). As the years went on, my medication regiment grew, I had a bout with four bleeding ulcers in my stomach, and was prescribed a medication to help in preventing future problems with ulcers. Then as the years went on, my blood pressure became an issue, it was beginning to get out of control, to the point, that I had three different medication prescribed to help in lowering my blood pressure, but about a decade ago, I was taking three medications, plus a patch to help with the control of my blood pressure, and now in the last five years, I am back down to two meds. My medication continues to be substituted for another medication, for one reason or another. And like I mentioned in my first book, "My Renal Life" (I know it, I live it), I know medication isn't perfect, and I am a setting example of that, for the last decade, I have had medicine changed, substituted for another, decreased, increased, stopped, restarted, and rotated to every other day, pills almost cut to much of nothing, (because the dose that I may have to take, it doesn't by chance come in that particular dosage, that is required), you name it, I've experienced it all. I know when it comes to taking antibiotics,

I tend to have some side effects, that truly becomes a struggle for me, like for instance - antibiotics can decrease my appetite, significantly, and I also have trouble with plummeting blood pressure, these side effects do become a problem with my health, while taking antibiotics, in which most cases, antibiotics are prescribed for seven to even two weeks of usage. This is what I did to try to remedy these problems that I have with taking antibiotics. First, because of my very unhealthy appetite, I am aware that I don't get enough protein in my diet, so to remedy that, and keep in mind, I really don't have an appetite, I practically have to make myself eat something. I would make a homemade egg flower soup, and put plenty of egg whites in it, because one large egg white, contains 3.5 grams of protein, I drop three egg whites in the liquid. Here is my recipe for Egg Flower Soup.

Ingredients: 3 large eggs whites, 2 cups chicken broth, 1 cup green onion - finely chopped, ½ cup - carrots - cut into small cubes, ½ cup - celery - cut in small cubes, and ½ cup - shallots - thinly sliced, 1 tsp - Mrs. Dash table blend, 1 tsp - pepper, 1 tsp - salt, 1 tsp - rice wine vinegar, 1 tbsp - minced ginger, and the zest and Juice of half a lemon, and 1 tsp - minced garlic, and 1 tbsp - extra virgin olive oil

Instructions: In a saucepan, over medium heat, saute in olive oil - green onions, shallots, carrots, celery, ginger and garlic, until the vegetables are tender, then add the lemon zest, and then the chicken broth, rice wine vinegar, bring to a boil, then add the dry seasonings - Mrs. Dash, pepper, and salt. Dropped the egg whites a little at a time, in the boiling broth, oh make sure you use low sodium chicken broth, so that you can control the amount of salt to add to it. I add about 1 tsp of salt, but that is your preference, especially if you are a patient that don't have issues with high levels of sodium in your body. Glo's tip: to try to get as much of the protein that you can, try to eat all of the egg whites. The vegetables are low biological protein, and the vegetables won't give you as much protein intake. Also, hemo patients, if you have issues with fluid overload, try not drinking much of the broth, because it will help to keep the fluid intake in check.

Getting back to medication, which is another very important aspect of maintaining good health with dialysis. Even though following a proper renal diet, eating the right foods, the right amount and if necessary, avoiding some foods all together, which mean knowing your limits, plays a very important part in following a proper renal diet, medication also helps in keeping the minerals in your body, in normal range. So, taking medication as prescribed is a plus, in accomplishing this, but I am here to tell you, that taking medication can be complicated as well, I remember there was this one time, in the early days of dialysis, when I was admitted to the hospital from ER, I didn't take any of my medication, for almost a whole day, and at the time, I ask my doctor, why hadn't I had any of my medication, and he told me, not to worry, because I only missed one dose, but I was told when I started taking a certain medication, try not to miss any of it. Learning this, I don't panic, when I may miss a dose for some reason or another. It is funny to me, how changing or being assigned a new doctor, some of what a patient has been following while under the medical attention of another doctor, especially for a significant amount of time, and all of a sudden, when you change or assigned a new doctor, for one reason or another, and in my case, I was assigned a new neprologist, because of the choosing of a certain insurance. Being assigned this new neprologist, became very beneficial to me. My new neprologist, carefully examined my records, and immediately was alarmed at how high my PTH levels were, and he couldn't understand why I didn't have my thyroid glands, surgically removed, because it was the most logical solution to this problem. He immediately scheduled to have my glands removed, and ever since then, it has been a decade now, my PTH levels are most of the time staying steady in normal range, but on occasion, it gets a little elevated, and my meds are quickly adjusted. I do believe in my opinion, that there wasn't a great deal known about the effects of the PTH level, where dialysis is concerned. My previous neprologist just kept changing and rotating my vitamin D med, with no success. I really don't know from this day, if I would have never been assigned a new neprologist, that I would eventually have this surgery to remove my thyroid glands. Go Figure! That is what makes this so complicated, with decisions and solutions. Now about my binders, I remember when I first started dialysis, I was prescribed phos los to help in binding the foods, before it could reach my bloodstream, but with pho lo, I began to have issues with my calcium levels, and then I was prescribed a new phosphorus binder, which helped to bind the foods, and also keep my calcium levels in check. All in all, medicine can effect your health in general, as I even have had medication that would cause my lips to swell up. I have had many allergic reactions to certain meds prescribed, especially varies antibiotics, which I would break out in a rash, or closing of my throat, body sweats, chills and shakes, and of course, uncontrollable itching. However, through the years of dialysis, I discovered I am allergic to a number of medicines. I can't even take the standard antibiotics for peritonitis, I always have to seek medical attention from the Emergency Department. When you are prescribed a new medication by your doctor, ask him what it is for, and how long do you have to take this particular medication, because some medication are only taken temporary, until the problem is solved, and because we are dialysis patients, some meds prescribed, have to be taken as long as you are a dialysis patient. However, when I received the blessing of my first cadaver kidney transplant, I stopped taking just about all the meds that I was taking while I was a dialysis patient, but there was a great deal more medication taking with a transplant, which I was told that the medication will taper down as the months and years went by with the transplanted kidney. If you started reading this book from the beginning, then you have read about my transplant experience and meds that was prescribed.

A recap of what a blessing dialysis has been to me, and how technology, continues to find ways to help people with kidney disease, live a long productive life:

As the months and years went by, dialysis treatment began to become a little easier, I learned to incorporate it into my personal life, and I also began to accept what is inevitable in my life. I look back at how advance dialysis treatment has become since my father's days on dialysis. The dialyzer has changed tremendously, back in the day when my father would do home treatment, the machine sort of look like a big tank, in which he would have to use the outside hose to run water into the machine, and he would also have to do his chemical testing himself. My mom also played an important part in the dad's treatment, she was sort like his personal nurse, she would take his vitals before inserting the needles in his forearm. Everything is so different with dialysis today, my dad was on dialysis treatment for six hours, three days a week. I in the beginning was undergoing treatment for two and half hours. But four years ago, going back to hemo dialysis treatment temporarily, I was on dialysis three and half hours, three days a week, due to the fact that I had a catheter in my groin, in which the flow is only 300, when most patients with grafts and fistulas run at around 400 or 450. The second time around, I observed how face the little wheel was turning other fellow patients dialyzer, when my was barely going around in a circular motion. Your weight also becomes a factor as to how long you have to dialysis at each treatment and how much kidney function that you have remaining. Your treatment can run very smooth, if you listen to the tips that I'm about to reveal to you. They will become very important in the maintaining of your health between treatments.

1. Become involved in your treatment, ask questions about your dialyzer and what are the purpose of the numbers on the display panel, a tech or nurse will be happy to answer any of your questions. During my father's time on dialysis, these machines weren't in existence, today we have an advantage of knowing what everything means, and how it effects our treatment.

2. Regarding your weight, it is a very important factor in maintaining your health between treatments, and if you do learn this in the beginning, you will soon become very knowledgeable about what keeps you healthy and having a smooth treatment.

3. Your dietitian will become a very important part in maintaining your health also, she will from time to time hand out flyers about your diet, what to eat? And what not to eat? Moderation is an important word to learn when it come to your diet. I know in the past before dialysis came into play, you could practically eat just about anything, but that's not the case anymore, now that you are a dialysis patient. What becomes important is your labs and how to keep your values in range, I know it can be a little difficult to maintain this between treatments, but you'll soon learn. If you don't follow a renal diet, you could develop other problems with your lungs, heart, etc. etc. Your sodium becomes a factor, because too much salt in your diet, could result to hypertension or (high blood pressure as it is commonly referred as). Potassium is very important to maintaining your health on dialysis, because with a high potassium level your heart could be affected in a very serious way, causing heart disease or maybe a heart attack, that could result in undergoing bypass surgery. So please watch your cholesterol intake.

Here is a chart outlining your monthly nutrition report, it could vary at various units, but all in all the level ranges are about the same at every unit.

Albumin - The protein intake needs to be adequate to help prevent infections and aid in wound healing.
Goal - 4.0 or Higher

NPCR HD UKM - Maintaining good protein and calories in your diet
Goal - 1.0 or Higher

HCT CALC (HGBX3) - Maintaining good blood cell count. Always take your renal vitamin every day (Note: Remember to take your renal vitamin after treatment on dialysis days) to help maintain normal red blood cells.

Iron Saturation - Maintaining a good iron level. To prevent anemia. Remember to take your iron medication and in some cases IV iron could be given during dialysis treatment, but in some cases if the ferritin is high, you may not need IV iron administered.
Goal - 20 to 50%

Ferritin - Indicates your Iron stores.
Goal - 100 to 800

Calcium - Maintaining healthy bones
Goal - 8.4 to 10.2 - for non-dialysis patients
Goal - 8.4 to 9.5 - for dialysis patients

Phosphorus - To keep your bones and heart healthy. Very important to take your binders right before, during or right after your meal, and at snack time. The right amount will be prescribed to you during the initial beginning of dialysis treatment, However the amount could be changed if the phosphorus levels began to rise and are out of the normal range.
Goal - 3.5 to 5.5

PTH - Parathyroid Hormone Level - To maintain healthy bones
Goal - 150 to 300

Potassium - To keep your heart working well (meaning your muscles and nerves)
Goal - 3.5 to 5.5

Cholesterol - To keep the heart functioning well.
Goal - 100 to 200

Triglycerides - Fats found in your blood.
Goal - Below 200

Glucose - (Sugar) - Normal fasting blood sugar is 80 to 120. Note: Diabetics should keep there levels in this range at the beginning of the day, and below 160 about 2 hours after meals.
Goal - 80 to 160

KT/V TOTAL (F) - (The Adequacy of Dialysis) - It measures how well your blood is being cleaned
Results are affected by length of time on the machine, type of dialyzer used, blood flow rate, and access function. Remember stay on the machine for your entire treatment prescribed. With adequate dialysis treatment a patient feels better, have fewer hospitalizations and live longer.

Fluid weight gain between treatments is very important. NOTE: TOO MUCH FLUID WEIGHT CAN CAUSE HIGH BLOOD PRESSURE, SWELLING, SHORTNESS OF BREATH, AND MUSCLE CRAMPS DURING TREATMENT. Avoid salt, high sodium foods, and fast foods (scratch that, because that's asking a lot, just try to indulge only once in a while).

Fluid Intake:
Goal - 2 to 3 Kg or 3 to 5% of body weight between treatments.

Facts to take notice: High Blood Pressure is on the rise. African-Americans in particular have one of the highest rates of high blood pressure, not only in this country, but in the world as a whole. There are more and more people developing kidney disease because of uncontrolled blood pressure, and I've noticed in the last decade (at my dialysis unit), there are so many older teenagers and young adults undergoing dialysis of some kind, because of high blood pressure, diabetes and heart disease. And speaking of diabetes, the numbers are growing tremendously, because of obesity in this country. More and More children are developing type 2 diabetes, because of the overweight and obese problem.

Note: Although most of my recipes in this book are renal friendly and for a non-diabetic, like myself, there's still a concern for the diabetic dialysis patients. So please remember diabetics you must keep your glucose level between the range of 80-120 a the beginning of the day and below 160 about two (2) hours after meals.

I have learned that, anyone can be at increased risk for Type 2 Diabetes if you are: Overweight; Obese, over the age of 40, are African American, Hispanic, Native American, or Asian; Have a family history of type 2 diabetes; have predicaments (fasting blood glucose between 100 and 125 mg/dl); have high blood pressure (higher than 140/90 mm Hg); have low HDL (good) cholesterol less than 40 mg/dl) or high Triglycerides (more than 250 mg/dl); Non-active (no exercise) or little exercise; or you can develop diabetes during pregnancy.

Fact about a Type 2 Diabetes Diet:

People at risk for type 2 diabetes and those of you who already developed it, remember whole grains and fiber are beneficial, because they do not increase blood sugar and insulin as much as refined carbs, such as white bread and white rice.

A Second Invite Into Glo's Renal Friendly Kitchen

Understanding and following your diet will help keep you feeling healthy. As you will learn more, while following the renal diet, you will be able to include a wider variety of foods in your meals. I have included information to help you make decisions about your food intake. Including the food finder list for those very important minerals, (sodium, potassium, and phosphorus), you will soon discover, that keeping these very important minerals in normal range, could be very challenging at times, because of some of the restrictions, placed on various food groups. Although, I tried to list as many foods as I possibly can, if there isn't a particular meat, fruit, vegetable, or dairy product not mentioned, by all means, ask your dialysis unit dietitian to research it for you, before you venture into unknown territory. *Choose your food wisely* and just because you have to follow a renal diet, there are compromises to enhancing the flavor of various foods, without having all that sodium (salt) for a good taste. Try lemon and wine vinegars on your meats, main dishes and vegetable dishes. I also share what I have learned through the years about vinegar. I have tried my best to include the nutritional facts about the recipes that I share in this book, but some of the homemade recipes that I share, may not have all the nutritional values included, so make sensible food choices, for what is required for your particular renal diet, because every patients diet is unique in its on way. I have collected many renal friendly recipes, throughout my twenty plus years of dialysis. Also below are some tips I learned in my humble beginning of dialysis, that I would like to share with my readers.

For best results, use the following tips:

* **Read labels on foods carefully**
* **Avoid salt in any form (iodized salt, vegetable salt, sea salt, Or seasoning salts)**

* Avoid salt substitutes or "lite" salt
* Watch for sodium compounds in foods
* Watch for potassium compounds such as: Baking Powder Substitute, Potassium Chloride, Tartrate baking powders.
* Measure foods by weight or measurements as recommended For specific foods

Before checking out my recipes in Glo's Renal Friendly Kitchen, I would like to share some of my cooking tips, and ways of how I made most of my homemade recipes renal friendly, however, you will discover that most of the recipes in my book, will have nutritional facts included, which are recipes designed for a renal diet, in which I have been collecting since 1990, and I will also include some of my homemade recipes, that may not have nutritional facts, that relate to the renal diet, however, although some of the recipes will state the nutritional facts, it may not list how much phosphorus is in its contents.

Like I mentioned before born in New Orleans, and raised in Houma, La, I learned early on from my mom, how to prepare creole/cajun meals. Just about every dish that she would prepare, she would start out with a saute of (what was known in Louisiana as) holy trinity - (which consist of onions, bell pepper and celery). This combination would almost always be a part of a meal. And in some cases if it's a stew, gumbo or jambalaya, or just a nice pot of red beans and rice. Yes, red beans, we like our beans with a gravy, not watery, so a roux really makes those beans scream, Yum Yum! But remember dialysis patients when it comes to beans, we have to be careful of the phosphorus. I'm not telling you to take beans completely out your diet, because that's simply ridiculous, just don't overindulge O.K? Know your limits.

Before you check out my recipes, I'd like to share a few facts with you, about the seasonings and ingredients used for various dishes throughout the recipe section of this book.

Creole Seasoning, for instance - I use Creole seasoning to give various dishes better taste, this seasoning mixed with onion powder & garlic powder will enhance the flavors in whatever dish you cook, and besides I grew up on this seasoning. You could say it was a part of my creole heritage.

Facts about Creole Seasoning: This seasoning consist of salt, sugar, red pepper, black pepper, paprika, onion, garlic and spices. ¼ tsp serving contains 150 mg of sodium (salt). Glo's Tip: I use Creole seasoning in most of my dishes along with onion powder, and garlic powder. In most of the recipes I would mix (whisk) the dry seasonings together in a separate small bowl. I love seasoning my meats especially with Creole seasonings, however most of my cuisine is seasoned with Creole seasonings, I call this Glo's Special Enhancer - (Creole seasoning, onion powder, garlic powder) and sometime a little fresh ginger or nutmeg for that extra kick.

Remember sodium (salt) intake is a big issue with dialysis patients. Come now, I know and you know that you can't just eliminate salt in your diet all together, so let's compromise and limit our intake of sodium. If you have read the earlier discussions in this book, I mentioned some facts about sodium and it bares repeating. When it comes to purchasing foods with sodium as the content, these days whatever packaging that the food items comes in, in most cases it will almost always specify how much sodium is in its contents.

Check out the following ways that sodium is specified and how much milligrams is in its contents:

Sodium free - less than 5 mg of sodium
Reduced sodium - usual level of sodium reduced by 25%
Very low sodium - 35 mg of sodium
Light (lite) sodium - usual level of sodium reduced by 50%
Low sodium - 140 mg of sodium

Fact: Remember a dialysis patient can have about 2000 mg of sodium, a day, compared to a non-dialysis patient, who can eat twice as much as that a day.

Sometime I will purchase creole seasoning from a store, but when I'm in the mood, I make my own. If you are interested in making your own from scratch here is the recipe:

Creole Seasoning Blend:

Ingredients:

2 ½ tbsp sweet paprika
1 tsp salt
2 tbsp garlic powder   ***CREOLE SEASONING BLEND RECIPE***

2 tbsp onion power
1 tbsp cayenne pepper
1 tbsp dried oregano
1 tbsp dried thyme

Instructions: Mix (whisk) all these ingredients together and store in an air-tight container. You can store it for up to 2 ½ to 3 months.

I also use chicken broth to enhance the flavor of most of my dishes. I always use chicken broth that's 99% fat free. One (1) cup of chicken broth contains 840 mg of sodium (salt), but it's better to use low sodium broth, so that you can control the salt in your recipes. The calories are only 10 in a 1 cup serving.

Glo's Tip: I often coat the bottom of a glass casserole dish with broth (about 1 1/4 cups), worchestire sauce, (a few drops) a little red wine vinegar, (about 1 tsp.) garlic, onion and herbs (if necessary for blending the flavors), and Mrs. Dash (table blend). I use this blend mostly when I bake chicken, lean pork chops, shoulder steaks or lamb chops.

If you have End Stage Renal Disease, (like myself), being on dialysis, phosphorus intake in your diet is very serious also. I know we have to watch very carefully what we eat, and even though it is mandatory that the nutritional facts are explained on products these days, it will indicate how much sodium and maybe in some cases how much potassium, and fat content, but some of the products will indicate if some source of phosphorus is part of the content, but it won't specific how much phosphorus. Well to be honest with you, individuals that don't have any renal issues or dialysis issues don't need to be concerned about their phosphorus intake, like we do. Just make sensible food choices where the phosphorus is concerned, and by all means very importantly, don't forget to take your phosphorus binders prescribed.

Glo's Tip: Usually when I just want to cook some really tasty meat, I use my own special seasoning blend and wet ingredients in a glass casserole dish, with the oven preheated at 375 F. For about 4 lean pork chops, or 4 shoulder steaks, or even 4 lamb chops. First I would mix the wet ingredients in a bowl and then mix the dry seasoning in another bowl And pour the wet ingredients in the casserole dish, and season my meat with the dry seasoning and place the meat in the casserole dish and place in the oven and bake for 1 hour on one side and flip each piece of meat over for another maybe ½ hour more. This is a real simple way to cook the meat and to avoid cooking or frying the meat on the stove. Besides we need to watch the cholesterol. Right!

Remember to use low sodium chicken broth, so you can control the salt in your recipe

Wet ingredients:	*Dry ingredients:*
1 ½ cups - chicken broth	1 tsp - creole seasoning
1 ½ tsp - worchestire sauce	1 tbsp - onion powder
1 tsp - rice wine vinegar	1 tbsp - garlic powder
2 tbsp - white wine	1 tbsp - Mrs. Dash (table blend)

If you haven't really dabble with different seasonings, herbs and spices, here's a little list of some great seasonings to have on hand to help enhance the flavor of your recipes.

My favorite - creole seasoning, season salt, lemon pepper, pepper flakes, and Mrs. Dash - (table blend, garlic & herb, and Italian medley) - actually there are others that are great, but these are the main varieties that I use.

Herbs: dried - thyme, rosemary, basil, bay leaf, dill, mint and tarragon (if fresh is available, that's great to use also).

Spices: cumin, ginger, curry powder, onion powder, and garlic powder

Wine vinegars: white wine, red wine, balsamic, sherry, and champagne vinegar

Cooking wines: white, red, and sherry

Worchestire sauce, soy sauce, and teriyaki sauce

Facts About:

Onion Powder - 1 tbsp is equivalent to one (1) small size fresh onion
Garlic Powder - 1/8 tsp is equivalent to one (1) clove fresh garlic

Season all season salt - ½ tsp contains 240 mg of sodium, fat free, and no carbohydrates

Meat tenderizer - ¼ tsp contains 400 mg of sodium (use wisely- make sensible choices)

Creole seasoning - ¼ tsp contains 150 mg of sodium

Tarragon - brings a refreshing licorice like flavor to foods - it's classic with chicken and fish. It's great to add as a extra seasoning to breadcrumbs.

Basil leaves - an herb used to enhance the flavors in pasta, potatoes, macaroni salad, eggplant, carrots, cauliflower, zucchini, and yellow squash. - use 1 tsp for frozen vegetables and 2 tsp - for fresh vegetables

Thyme - an herb used in jambalaya, clam chowder, ground beef, especially for meat loaf, pasta, to enhance sauces, and shish-kabobs.

Glo's Tip: Use one (1) tsp for pasta, sauces and shish kabobs.

Mrs. Dash - makes a variety of seasonings and I thank God this was invented, because it is a dear friend to me as a dialysis patient, and if you haven't tried Mrs. Dash seasonings, I strongly suggest that you add this as a part of the flavoring to your many dishes, because you don't know what you are missing, it will very much enhance the flavor of your homemade cuisine and it is so very good for your health, with it's blend of savory herbs and spices. I use it all the time, as you will see in many of my homemade recipes that I share with you in this book.

Mrs. Dash - contains no sodium (salt), or MSG. It contains onion, black pepper, chili pepper, parsley, celery seed, basil, oregano, thyme, cayenne pepper, corainder, cumin, rosemary, garlic, lemon juice, red bell pepper, and oil of lemon. ¼ tsp contains 10 mg of K+ (potassium).

Glo's Tip: Add 1 tbsp of Mrs. Dash seasoning to your beef, chicken pork or fish recipes

Here's some measurements that maybe helpful to you, when preparing your meals:

1 tbsp = ½ ounce
2 tbsp = 1 ounce
½ cup = 4 ounces
1 cup = 8 ounces

1 ½ cup = 12 ounces (equivalent to a can of soda)
2 cup = 16 ounces = (1 pint)
4 cup = 32 ounces (1 quart)

FACTS: Apple Cider Vinegar can help to prevent high blood pressure. Back in the early 70's, my dad would drink apple cider vinegar everyday, and at the time I didn't know why he was drinking so much apple cider vinegar. Now that I've gotten older and head to face the drama of poly cystic kidney disease and dialysis, I soon found out by reading about vinegar, that it is very healthy for patient with renal kidney disease and besides it's also great as an added addition to salads and main dishes. It really enhances the flavor when used in many of my dishes.

When eating such foods as beans, you should only eat a ½ cup serving, because some of these foods contain a significant amount of phosphorus, potassium and or sodium.

I know most of us grew up on big pots of beans and rice, especially red beans, but being a dialysis patient you should limit your intake of these foods: also black-eyed peas, garbanzo, kidney, lentils, pinto and split pea.

Cheese (natural) - 1 ounce a day
Cold cuts - (mainly chicken or turkey breast) - 2 slices - (no ham or salami) PLEASE!!!
Cottage Cheese, (creamed/low fat) - only - ¼ cup
Peanut Butter - (2 tbsp)
Pizza, cheese - Be careful, just about all of us love pizza, (only 1 slice) PLEASE!!!, I know this is depriving us, isn't it. But I got to be real with you, I know you don't want to have one of those itching attack, that I repeatedly keep mentioning, that's no joke, I'm not kidding.

NOTE: Tofu, soft (½ cup), firm (¼ cup) - allowed for a dialysis patients intake

You must avoid anchovies, bacon (pork or Canadian), beef jerky, canned meats, cheese, (processed or spreads), chili, corn beef, crab (imitation), any cured meats such as ham or hot dogs, herring, kosher meats, liver, salt pork, sardines, and sausages. I guess you say, come now, this is going just a little too far. Just like I said previously, everything we like, is off limits. Just try to eat a little in moderation, I know it is impossible to just give up all these wonderful delectable. I must admit from time to time I have a little taste of off limit foods, just to feel normal. (laugh).

Glo's Tip: As you begin to try my recipes, refer to these nutritional facts from time to time, O.K? You may be rewarded with great lab results. And what does that mean?, and yes you are on the right track to maintaining good health between hemo dialysis treatment and everyday peritoneal dialysis treatment.

Glo's Tip: Gather all your ingredients first, that are mentioned in my recipes and then start your preparation, trust me this will make your cooking more organized and you will have a sense of better control in your kitchen.

I've never been a big breakfast person, and I know it is said to be the most important meal of the day. I usually eat a couple of boiled eggs without the yolk, to watch my cholesterol intake, and maybe some kind of fruit cut up and marinated with balsamic vinegar, to start my day.

NOTE: *For a individual who undergoes hemo dialysis treatment, usually the renal diet consist of low protein, low sodium, and low potassium, but there are cases where the patient, may need more protein, or more potassium in their diet, especially if they are peritoneal dialysis patients, their protein and potassium are always at question Because it can be easily removed during your hemo dialysis treatment and more can be removed during your nigh time treatment with peritoneal cycler treatment..*

Suggested Meal Plan For Renal Diet

Suggested Meal Plan:

Breakfast

Dairy List .... 1 serving
Fruit List..................... 1 serving
Fat List....................... 3 servings
Free List......................used as
Desired for calories

(Fruit List)
Bread/Starch List............ 2 serving

Sample Menu:

Breakfast

¾ cup - frost flakes cereal (Bread List)
½ cup - whole milk   (Dairy List)
1 slice toast   (Bread List)
Butter/margarine   (Fat List)
Jelly/Jam   Free List)
1 cup coffee or tea with Mocha Mix or Sugar
(to be used in limited quantities)½ cup - apple juice

Suggested Meal Plan:

Lunch:

Meat List........... 1 ½ serving
Bread/Starch...... 1 serving
Fruit List........... 1 serving
Vegetable List..... 1 serving
Fat List........... 3 servings
½ cup - vegetables
2 pear halves
7-UP

Dinner:

Meat List.......... 1 ½ ounces
Bread/Starch..... 2 servings
Vegetable List.... 1 serving
Fat List.......... 3 servings

Sample Menu:

Lunch:

½ roast beef sandwich made with:
1 slice bread   (Bread List)
1 ½ oz. Roast beef   (Meat List)
1 tbsp. Mayonnaise   (Fat List)
1 cup - unsalted soup
(Vegetable List)
(Fruit List)
(Free List)

Dinner:

1 ½ oz. Hamburger patty   (Meat List)
½ cup white rice   (Bread/Starch List)
½ cup asparagus   (Vegetable List)
1 slice bread   (Bread List)

Butter/margarine	*(Fat List)*
Lemonade or 7-UP	*(Free List)*
Hard Candy	*(Free List)*

Note: (if you need extra calories in your diet) - 1 cup coffee or tea (Misc. List) with sugar or Mocha Mix

FREE LIST:

Sweets (for extra calories) - be careful diabetes, make sensible food choices

Candy corn
Chewing gum
Cotton candy
Cranberry sauce
Fruit ice
Gum drops
Hard candy
Honey
Jam
Jelly
Jelly beans
Lollipops
Popsicles
Preserves
Sugar
Syrup

A reminder on the topics of:
Low Biological Protein vs. High Biological Protein:

Facts: These facts are mentioned in the chapter "What is Protein", but it bares repeating before you attempt to prepare any of my recipes in this book: Some of the Main Fare recipes will have an excessive amount of protein, but some of my dishes, especially the vegetable dishes have a small amount of protein, meaning (low biological protein), so you may need to add some meat, but in the case if you are a vegeterian, you may have to add some seafood or tofu to get the recommended amount of protein needed for that meal.

*Remember: Good quality protein (meaning **High Biological Protein**) is used more efficiently by the body and create fewer waste products. Such as egg, egg whites, fish, chicken, turkey, pork, lamb, beef, veal and tofu.*

*Vegetables, legumes, nuts, bread and starches are **Low Biological Protein**, and are not used as efficiently by the body. (SO PLEASE CHECK THE RECIPE FIRST TO MAKE SURE YOU WILL GET THE PROPER AMOUNT OF NUTRIENTS NEEDED TO MAINTAIN GOOD HEALTH BETWEEN HEMO TREATMENTS AND EVERYDAY PERITONEAL TREATMENTS, BECAUSE EVERY DIALYSIS PATIENT DIET IS UNIQUE, AND FROM TIME TO TIME, YOUR DIET WILL CHANGE .*

FOR EXAMPLE: YOUR MONTHLY LAB RESULTS WILL INDICATE HOW WELL YOU ARE DOING WITH YOUR RENAL DIET.

PROTEINS COULD BE LOW (ALBUMIN), OR YOUR POTASSIUM IS TOO HIGH OR IN SOME CASES MAY GET TOO LOW, BUT IN ANY CASE, THERE ARE SOLUTIONS TO THESE PROBLEMS,

A dialysis patient needs six to ten ounces of protein a day

Example: 3 ounces - hamburger patty	3 ounces - pork chop
4 ounces - beef steak - 3"x4"	2 ounces - shrimp (5 med size)
3 ounces - fish fillet - 3"x3"	1 ounces - one egg (whole)
3 ounces - ½ chicken breast	2 ounces - egg whites

One small serving of phosphorus a day
        Example: ½ cup milk   1 oz. - cheese

Albumin - two to three meals and one to two snacks a day to get enough protein and calories

Vegeterian need two to three ounces of tofu - Example: one soy burger
A dialysis patient shouldn't have but 2,000 milligrams of sodium a day - compared to most people who eat twice as much. (to keep blood pressure from elevating).

The list below is the ounces recommended for dialysis patients - (note: for the seafood category the servings are equivalent to a 1 ounce serving. This little list can assist you when measuring your meat for protein intake.

Beef, fresh, - 4 ounces = 3"x4"
Chicken, breast - 3 ounces = ½
Cottage cheese, dry (¼ cup)
Duck - 3 ounces
Egg (1 whole) - 1 ounce
Egg (2 egg whites) - 1 ounce
Egg substitute (¼ cup)
Fish, fillet - 3 ounces - 3"x3"
Lamb - 3 ounces

Egg substitute - (¼ cup)
Fish, fillet - 3 ounces - 3'x3"
Lamb - 3 ounces
Pork, fresh - 3 ounces
Rabbit - 3 ounces

Nutritional Facts:

A one (1) ounce serving of each of the meats and seafood (as indicated below) averages:

Protein - 8 grams
Sodium - 30 mg
Potassium - 100 mg

Phosphorus - 70 mg
Calcium - 10 mg
Calories - 60

Turkey, fresh, or frozen
Veal

Venison

Seafood:
Clams (3 medium size)
Oysters (3 med. Size)
Crabmeat (¼ cup)
Scallops (3 large size)
Lobster meat (¼ cup)
Shrimp (3 large size)

Remember a dialysis patient needs about 8 to 11 ounces per day of protein foods

Glo's Tip: I invested in a food scale, to measure my meat. Weigh your meats cooked, without the bone. Remember four (4) ounces of raw meat is equivalent to three (3) ounces of meat cooked.

Chicken:

1 chicken wing - equivalent to - one (1) ounce of protein
1 chicken thigh - equivalent to - two (2) ounces of protein
1 small chicken breast or one small pork chop - equal - three (3) ounces of protein - (this would be about the size of a deck of cards)
1 large chicken breast - equivalent to four (4) ounces of protein

All about Vinegar
(tips on using vinegar in cooking and nutritional facts)

Vinegar, has been a staple in my family for a long time, especially when I started dialysis. I learned a great deal from my mom, and other family members, like the home remedies that they passed on about vinegar. Now, let me share some of those home remedies with you. Because of PD treatment, I became very skeptic about cleanliness, I would keep my garbage disposal, clean and fresh-smelling, by making vinegar cubes. I mixed one cup of vinegar in a sufficient of water to fill an ice tray, then freeze the mixture and run the cubes through the disposal. After the grinding action has stopped, flush with cold water for a minute or so. I also use vinegar to disinfect my dishwasher drain, I add ½ cup of white wine vinegar to the rinse cycle.

I make a marinade, for meat, by using ½ cup of red wine vinegar and dissolve a beef bouillon cube in a cup, which makes a great meat tenderizer.

I also use red wine vinegar to marinade my beef, pork and lamb, and when I want a marinade for poultry, seafood or vegetables, I use white wine vinegar instead. Tarragon white wine is great for fish. I always add a tsp of worchestire sauce for flavor to my marinade.

When I make rice, I add a tsp of white vinegar to the boiling water, which makes my rice fluffy and white.

When my lettuce is slightly wilted, I soak them in vinegar and water, to make them crispy once again.

Because we are living some very tough economic times, keeping the produce and any food from going bad too soon, I have come up with some tricks in accomplishing just that, of course, cheese, should be limited in the renal diet, I still purchase cheese on occasion, and to make it last, I wrap the block of cheese in some cheese cloth, slightly dampened in some white vinegar and sealing it in a air tight container, it last for several weeks.

Now, to boil a perfect egg, I add a tbsp of vinegar to the water, which prevents the whites from leaking out of a cracked egg. I hate this, when I am making deviled eggs. Even when I poach egg, I add a tsp of vinegar to the water to prevent separation.

Since, becoming a peritoneal dialysis patient, I am very skeptic of germs, so I use vinegar all over my kitchen to clean, my microwave oven, the cutting board, and meat cutting board.

Vinegar Tips for Cooking

Apple cider vinegar - It has a sweet and tangy flavor - I add it to soups, and varies vegetables such as - collard greens, cabbage, and okra

Balsamic vinegar - Is also sweet and very flavorful - I drizzle a little on fruits such - blackberries, strawberries, raspberries and blue berries, with a little cream topping

Malt vinegar - It has a very deep flavor, which is made from barley malt extract - I add this vinegar to fish, potato salad, pasta salad, and cole slaw

Red wine vinegar - It is very robust, and has low sodium - I use it to marinate steak, I also add it to beef stew, my homemade tomato sauce recipe, homemade Italian dressing recipe,

Rice wine vinegar - I use this vinegar in my stir fry dishes, shrimp fried rice, and okra creole recipe, because it is a very mild and sweet tasting vinegar

Tarragon flavored white wine vinegar - I use this vinegar to marinade chicken, and I also use it when I make veal

Pasta Dishes

FYI: Facts about Pasta and Vinegar

Pasta with vinegar, garlic, onions, and olive oil is a healthy meal. Pasta is low in fat and sodium and has just about 200 calories per 2-ounce serving - about 1 cup. Pasta is also a good source of fiber. ***Note: Fiber can stabilize blood sugar levels.*** Pasta is also high in nutrition values, containing calcium, iron, magnesium and protein.

The following pasta dishes are very healthy and quite easy to make. I make it very often to accompaniment many of my meat recipes, as well as seafood recipes too.

EASY CLAM LINGUINE

Ingredients:

1 lb. Linguine
4 cans baby clams, drained and rinsed
1 onion, thinly sliced
½ cup - shallots - chopped
3 clove - garlic - minced
¼ cup - extra virgin olive oil
1 tbsp - Mrs. Dash (table blend) seasoning
½ cup - chives

1 cup - white wine
½ cup - fresh chopped parsley
½ cup - fresh chopped basil
1 tsp - creole seasoning
1 tbsp - garlic powder
1 tbsp - onion powder
½ - lemon - zest & juice
½ - salt

Instructions:

In a pot with boiling water, add ½ tsp. Salt and pasta. Let boil for about 10 minutes until al dente. Strain well and add sauce to pasta.

To make the sauce, heat olive oil and onions, shallots, & garlic in large saute pan over medium heat. Saute onions, shallots & garlic until translucent. Add baby clams, and slowly add the wine to the pan, the parsley, basil & lemon zest & juice. Add Mrs. Dash, creole seasoning, garlic and onion powder and reduce heat and simmer for 10 minutes.

Add Pasta to the Clam Sauce mixture and toss. Garnish with chives.

Nutritional Facts: (based on a ½ cup serving)

This dish has about 208 calories, carbohydrates - 26g, protein - 15g, fat, 5g, sodium - 86mg, Potassium - 189mg, and phosphorus 167mg

EASY TO PREPARE COUSCOUS

Ingredients:

½ cup - shallots - finely chopped
½ tsp - margarine or extra virgin
Olive oil
1 cup - low-sodium chicken broth
2/3 cup - dry couscous

Cooking Instructions:

Saute chopped onion in the margarine or olive oil until tender. In a medium saucepan bring broth to a boil. Stir in couscous and onions. Let stand 5 minutes. Fluff lightly with fork before serving.

Nutrition Facts:

This side dish has about 115 calories, protein - 3.5g, fat - 2g, very low sodium about 24 mg, potassium 61mg, and phosphorus - 22mg, (even though the phosphorus is low, stick with your binder regiment prescribed) - please take your binders, I guarantee you won't regret it. Itch, Itch - need I say more.

ORZO W/ VEGETABLES & HERBS

Ingredients:

1 ½ cups dry orzo pasta
3 quarts water or low-sodium
Broth (for more flavor, if you Prefer)
2 tsp - garlic powder & onion powder
½ tsp - Italian seasoning
½ tsp - creole seasoning
1 tbsp - grated parmesan cheese
1 tsp - rice wine vinegar
½ cup - finely chopped - carrots
½ cup - finely chopped - celery
½ cup - sliced - shallots
½ cup - fresh chopped - cilantro
½ cup - fresh chopped - parsley

Cooking Instructions:

First bring 3 quarts of water or broth to a boil. Add orzo pasta to water or broth and stir. Return to a boil and cook, covered 10 to 12 minutes. Remove from heat and drain well in colander. Pour drained pasta into serving bowl. Add olive oil, garlic powder, onion powder, Italian seasoning, creole seasoning, and parmesan cheese. Toss gently and add the chopped vegetables and herbs and mix well.

Nutrition Facts: (facts based on a ½ cup serving)

There's about 137 calories in this dish, protein - 6.5g, low sodium about 20 mg, low potassium about 76mg, fat content - 3g, and most importantly about 92 mg of phosphorus, (but it's still important to take your binders as prescribed)

SPAGHETTI W/SHRIMP & MUSHROOMS CAJUN STYLE

Ingredients:

1 lb. Boiled med-size shrimp
1 finely chopped onion
2 garlic clove minced   *Note: Dialysis patients remember to*
1 tbsp butter or margarine   *watch your potassium intake, there*
1 ½ tbsp extra virgin olive oil   *is tomatoes in this recipe*
1 can of chopped tomatoes (14 oz.)
1 cup of tomato sauce
1 cup of chicken broth
1 tbsp tomato paste
1 small can of mushroom stems or 1 ½ cup of fresh mushrooms, sliced
1 tbsp Creole seasoning
1 tbsp onion powder
1/8 tsp garlic powder
1 tbsp chopped parlsey

Instructions:

Cook Spaghetti (according to package directions), in butter and olive oil saute onion and garlic for two minutes, stirring until soft.

Add tomato sauce and paste - bring to a boil. Reduce heat and boil rapidly, for five minutes. Stir in mushrooms sprinkle in creole seasoning, onion powder, and garlic powder. Cook for 2 minute.

Add chopped tomatoes, tomato sauce, broth and boiled shrimp. Cook for 2 minutes.

Meanwhile, drain spaghetti and return to pan. Pour the shrimp, mushroom sauce over the spaghetti and Sprinkle parsley on top and Serve.

Remember Dialysis pts. There is tomatoes in this dish (watch your potassium intake O.K!)

Main Fare

The main fare is very important to the renal diet, and there are issues with protein in the renal diet. Some patients may have to watch the protein in their renal diet, and there are some, especially, the peritoneal dialysis patients, that lose protein more easier with PD treatment, may need to add extra protein to their diet, but if that is not accomplished, a protein supplement could be prescribed to help in meeting their protein needs for their renal diet. Now, being that I have been on dialysis for almost two decades, I have experienced both sectors of the protein intake, and I know first hand how my PD treatment, keeps my protein intake in question, there are times when I may have to take a protein supplement to meet my protein needs with my renal diet, but all in all, when you get your monthly lab report, the report will indicate if you are eating enough protein, or if you need to add more protein to your diet, and maybe you may need to add a protein supplement, or if you are already prescribed protein supplement, to resume taking protein supplements, which can be a protein bar, protein drink, or maybe whey protein powder, that could be added to your meals or a homemade smoothie, which I will share some high protein smoothie recipes later on in this book. It is important to eat the high biological protein from your plate, first just in case, you get full very quick, like I do. Remember **High Biological Protein**, which is a very important part of the renal diet, in which this type of protein is good quality proteins, and are used more efficiently by the body and create fewer waste products, therefore, it is important that most of the protein in your renal diet come from good quality proteins, such as: eggs and egg whites, fish, chicken, turkey, pork, lamb, beef, veal and tofu.

The second type of protein, which is referred to as **Low Biological Protein** (low biological protein), and this is because one or more essential amino acids are missing. The body uses lower quality protein less effectively than high quality proteins. Vegetables, legumes, nuts, breads and other starches contain lower quality protein.

Remember both high and low quality proteins will be included in your healthy diet, but **Note: Some protein foods need to be limited due to high potassium and/or phosphorus contents.** *Just be more aware of these particular contents in foods, know your limits, and stick to them, as much as possible. I know from my own experience, that this is easier said than done, but try to as best as you can.*

Seafood: I very much like all kinds of seafood and an assortment of fish. Besides, born in New Orleans and raised in Houma, La., I grew up on seafood and fish, and I would like to share some of my favorite seafood and fish recipes, that I have accommodated to fit a renal diet. They are however, very easy to prepare and cook. Check these recipes out, on the following page.

Seared Breaded Sea Scallops
Broiled Lobster Cocktail
Broiled Salmon Fillet
Snow Crabs w/Tartar Sauce
Baked Salmon Fillet
Rosemary Roasted Salmon
Herbal Skillet Cod
Shrimp Scampi
Baked Tilapia w/Brown Butter

Chicken: In these economic times, chicken can be very affordable, and of course, chicken is a great source of protein for a renal diet, I will share with you some of my chicken recipes, following the seafood recipes.

Chicken and vegetables Cacciatora
Lemon Smothered Chicken Legs
Kickin Chicken Fajitas
Simple Roasted Chicken
Chicken and Pasta Dish

Turkey: Is another great and affordable source of protein, check out my easy to make turkey recipes

Turkey Salad with Balsamic Vinegarette
Turkey Meat Loaf

Pork: The other white meat, and another wonderful source of protein

Peppered Pork Tenderloin
Smothered Pork Chop

Beef: A great source of protein

Braised Beef w/ Mushroom Sauce
Chicken Fried Steak w/ Mushroom Sauce
Simple T-bone Grilled Steak
Easy & Simple Comfort at Home
Beef Stew

Lamb: Great source of protein

Lamb Skewers w/Dilled Lemon Sauce

Veal: Great source of protein

Veal Cutlets w/Herb Crust

Tofu:

Pasta Primavera Salad w/Tofu

SEARED BREADED SEA SCALLOPS

Ingredients:

12 large sea scallops　　　　　½ tsp dried oregano
½ tsp chili powder　　　　　　1 tsp creole seasoning
½ tsp cumin　　　　　　　　　1 tsp Mrs. Dash table blend
½ tsp season salt　　　　　　　1 tbsp each garlic powder and onion powder
2 tbsp olive oil　　　　　　　　¼ tsp black pepper
½ cup Italian bread crumbs, or plain bread crumbs, if you prefer

Instructions:

First, dry scallops well with paper towels, and then set aside. Second, in a small bowl, mix together chili powder, cumin, oregano, season salt, creole seasoning, Mr. Dash seasoning, garlic powder, onion powder, and black pepper. Third, season scallops on both sides with the dry seasoning mixture. Fourth, dust scallops lightly with the bread crumbs of your choice

Heat oil in a large skillet over high heat. Do not crowd scallops, cook three or four at a time. Sear scallops just until opaque, for about three (3) minutes per side. Serve warm.

Oh Wow! I love scallops, here are the nutritional facts - keep in mind, although scallops are a good source of protein, be aware of the excessive amount of phosphorus, that scallops contain, these nutritional facts are based on a 3 oz. Serving equivalent to about six large scallops

Calories - 125

Protein - 6 large cooked - 16.8 grams

Sodium - 135 mg

Potassium - 150 mg

Phosphorus - 203 mg

Fat - 8 grams

Sat Fat - 1 gram

Cholesterol - 30 mg

Carbohydrates - 1 gram

Fiber - 0 gram

Omega-3 - 0g

Glo's tip: I usually accompany my scallops, with a chilled vegetable orzo salad, along with some steamed broccoli florets, (these recipes are also included in this cookbook section of my book)

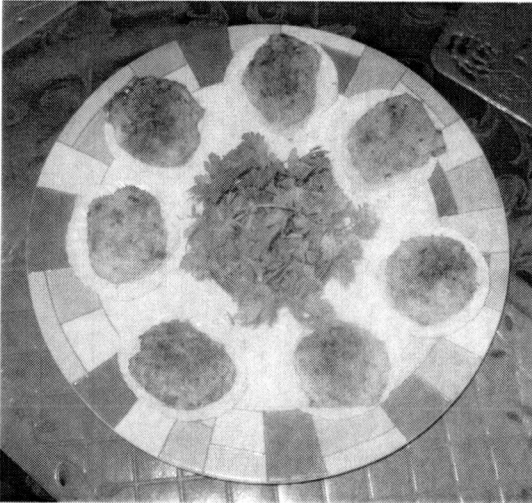

BROILED LOBSTER COCKTAIL

Ingredients:

2 (6 oz.) lobster tails
1 tbsp melted tub margarine
4 tsp fresh lime juice
1 tsp finely grated lime zest
1 tsp season salt
1 tsp black pepper
2 tsp - olive oil

½ tsp prepared horseradish
½ med. Avocado, peeled, pitted & diced
1/3 cup fresh or jarred mango - diced
1 tbsp finely chopped red onion
1 tbsp both of garlic and onion powder
Mrs. Dash (table blend)

Instructions:

Coat grill rack with nonstick cooking spray. Preheat grill to medium-high direct heat 350 to 400 degrees. Blend butter and 2 tsp - lime juice in a small bowl. Split underside of lobster shells lengthwise with kitchen scissors or sharp knife. Brush melted butter over the meat of lobster, sprinkle lightly salt, pepper, garlic powder, onion powder and table blend seasoning over the meat.

Place lobster, split side up, on grill. Grill, covered 5 minutes. Turn lobster, grill 3 to 5 minutes more or until meat is opaque. Remove from grill, set aside to cool slightly.

Meanwhile, in a medium bowl, blend oil, remaining 2 tsp - lime juice, lime peel and horseradish. Add avocado, mango and onion, toss to coat. Remove lobster from shells, discard shells. Cut lobster into bite-size chunks.

Spoon avocado mixture into large martini glasses or serving dishes. Top with lobster chunks.

Glo's tip: Serve your lobster cocktail with wedges of lime, if desired

Nutritional Facts:

Calories - 335	Sodium - 530mg	Cholesterol - 105mg
Protein - 27g	Carbohydrates - 16g	Omega - 3- 0g
Fat - 19g	Fiber - 5g	
Sat fat - 5g	1 oz - lobster - potassium - 51mg	

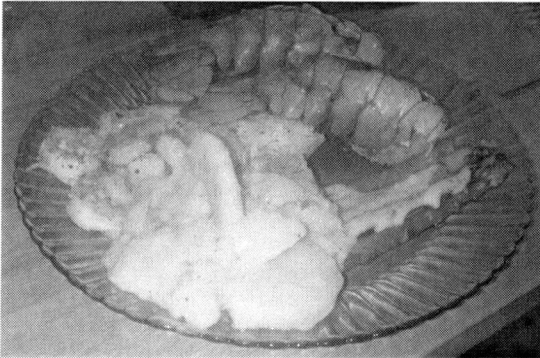

SNOW CRABS WITH HOMEMADE TARTAR SAUCE

Ingredients:

¾ cup - mayonnaise
¼ cup - fresh lime juice
2 tbsp - pickles - chopped
2 tbsp - red onions - chopped
1 tbsp - garlic powder
1 tbsp - onion powder
1 Obay seasoning bag

2 tbsp - fresh parsley - chopped
1 tsp - fresh jalapeno - chopped
¼ cup - olive oil
3 lbs - snow crabs
¼ tsp - salt
¼ tsp - black pepper
1 ½ cup - broth and water

Instructions: (Homemade tartar sauce recipe) -

Combine mayonnaise, lime juice, pickles, onion, parsley and jalapeno in medium bowl. Cover and refrigerator, until the crab is cooked.

In a large pot, season water and broth with garlic powder, onion powder, lime juice, salt, pepper, and drop Obay seasoning bag in the pot, set to boil for about five minutes, remove the crab and place on a platter, serve w/ homemade tartar sauce.

Nutritional Facts: (for 1 oz serving of crab)

Protein - 8g
Sodium - 30mg
Potassium - 100mg
Phosphorus - 70mg
Calcium - 10mg
Calories - 595
Fat - 32g
Sat Fat - 5g
Cholesterol - 275mg
Carbohydrates - 13g
Fiber - 0g
Omega - 3 - 2g

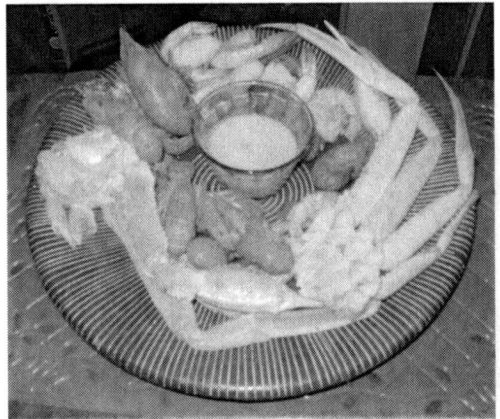

BAKED SALMON FILLET

Ingredients:

6 fillets or 3 lb. salmon - cut into six pieces, trimmed & skin removed
Juice of 1 lemon
¼ cup - olive oil
½ onion - sliced
1 lemon - thinly sliced
½ tsp - salt
¼ tsp - pepper

Instructions:

Preheat oven to 350 degrees. Cut 1 (16 in. long) sheet of aluminum foil for each fillet. Set aside.

Combine lemon juice, oil, salt and pepper, mix well. Brush the lemon juice mixture on both sides of the fillets.

Place each fillet toward 1 end of foil sheet. Place a couple of slices of onion and 1 slice of lemon on top. Fold foil to enclose fish, and seal to form a packet. Place packets on a large baking sheet with sides.

Bake 10 minutes (more if fillets are thick), or until fish flakes easily with a fork. Remove from oven; let packets stand unopened for five minutes. Open packets, reserving cooking juices. Place fillets on individual plates. Top with lemon slices and serve immediately.

Nutritional Facts:

Calories - 320
Fat - 16g
Sat Fat - 3g
Cholesterol - 115g
Sodium - 105mg
Protein - 42g

Phosphorus - 234mg
Omega - 3 - 2g
Carbohydrates - 2g
Fiber - 0g

ROSEMARY ROASTED SALMON

Ingredients:

4 (6 oz.) - salmon steaks
½ tsp - salt
3 lemons, thinly sliced

¼ cup - olive oil
¼ tsp - black pepper
¼ cup - fresh rosemary chopped

Instructions:

Preheat oven to 400 degrees. Place salmon on a large baking pan, coated with nonstick cooking spray. Drizzle with olive oil and season with salt and pepper. Top with lemon slices and chopped rosemary.

Roast salmon - 10 to 12 minutes or until fish flakes with fork. Garnish with fresh rosemary sprigs, if desired.

Nutritional Facts: Based on a 6 oz serving

Calories - 362
Fat - 23g
Sat Fat - 4g
Cholesterol - 80mg
Sodium - 360mg
Potassium - 1050mg
Carbohydrates - 13g
Fiber - 6g
Sugar - 2g
Protein - 32g
Omega - 3 - 2g

HERBAL SKILLET COD

Ingredients:

4 (6 oz.) fresh cod
8 tsp - olive oil, divided
¼ - red onion - thinly sliced (optional)
4 plum tomatoes, chopped
¼ cup - sliced black and green olives
Pinch - dried thyme, crushed

salt and pepper to taste
1 tsp. - Mrs. Dash
(table blend seasoning)
1 tsp - dried basil, crushed

Instructions:

Rinse fish, pat dry with paper towels. Season fish with salt, pepper, and Mrs. Dash table blend.

In a large skillet, heat 4 tsp of oil over medium heat. Add fish and (if desired) red onion. Cook 1 minute, turning once.

Top fish with tomatoes, olives and thyme. Reduce heat, cover and cook 2 minutes.

Drizzle with remaining 4 tsp oil, sprinkle with basil, cook, covered 2 to 3 minutes more or until fish flakes easily with a fork.

Nutritional Facts:

Calories - 245   Fiber - 1g   Carbohydrates - 3g
Fat - 12g   Protein - 31g   Sodium - 170mg
Sat Fat - 2g   Omega - 3 - 0g   Cholesterol - 75mg

Note: Atlantic cod - has about 117mg of phosphorus - based on a 3 oz serving - which falls in the lowest category of phosphorus

Pacific cod - 3 oz serving - 190mg of phosphorus - which falls in the highest category of phosphorus

BAKED TILAPIA WITH BROWN BUTTER

Ingredients:

1 ¼ lb - Tilapia fillets
1 tbsp - lemon juice
1 tbsp - tub margarine
1 tbsp - almonds, sliced and toasted

salt and pepper to taste
1 tsp. Mrs. Dash (herb and garlic) seasoning

Instructions:

Preheat oven to 350 degrees. Coat baking dish with nonstick cooking spray.

Season tilapia with salt, pepper, and Mrs. Dash (herb and garlic) seasoning. Drizzle with lemon juice. Place in a prepared baking dish. Bake 12 to 15 minutes or until fish flakes easily with a fork.

Meanwhile, melt margarine in a small skillet over low heat, until foamy and begins to brown, about 3 to 4 minutes. Strain margarine into a small bowl.

Drizzle margarine over tilapia, sprinkle with toasted almonds.

Nutritional Facts: based on a 3 oz serving of tilapia

Calories - 180
Fat - 7g
Sat Fat - 3g
Cholesterol - 80mg
Protein - 28g

Potassium - 15mg
Carbohydrates - 1g
Fiber - 0g
Sugar - 0g

Note: a 2 oz serving of almonds - contains 312mg of phosphorus, which falls in the highest category of phosphorus, also 2 oz serving of almonds has about 12.1g of protein - which falls in the highest category of protein.

SHRIMP SCAMPI

Ingredients:

1 ½ lb. shrimp
5 garlic cloves, chopped
½ cup - tub margarine
½ cup - white wine

Instructions:

Peel shrimp. Saute garlic in margarine, then add shrimp and cook until the shrimp turn pink.

Add wine and cook down (3 -5 minutes).

Serve over pasta or rice (follow package directions for both)

Nutritional Facts: based on a ½ cup serving

Calories - 265
Protein - 24g
Fat - 17g
Carbohydrates - 1g
Fiber - 0g
Sodium - 412mg
Potassium - 238mg
Calcium - 55mg
Phosphorus - 166mg
Cholesterol - 263mg

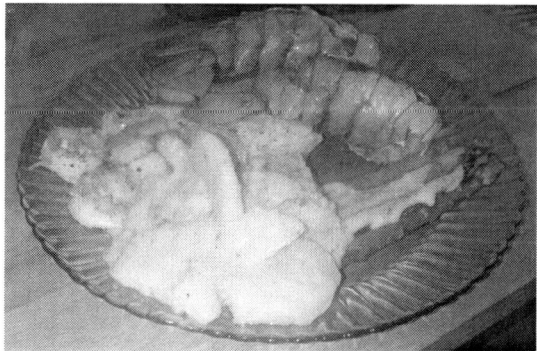

SHRIMP FRIED RICE

Ingredients:

3 tbsp - canola or peanut oil
½ cup - med. Size shrimp
¾ cup onion, diced
¾ tsp - black pepper
1 garlic clove, minced
1 tbsp - fresh ginger, minced

3 tbsp - scallions, chopped
1 cup - frozen peas and carrots
2 tbsp - canola or peanut oil
4 eggs, beaten
4 cups - white long grain rice
¼ tsp - salt

Instructions:

1. Preheat a large non-stick skillet over medium-high heat. Add 1 tbsp of oil.
2. Add onion and ½ tsp - black pepper and cook until onion is tender, about 2 minutes.
3. Add the garlic, ginger and scallions and stir for about 1 minute.
4. Add shrimp and stir frequently until heated.
5. Add peas and carrots and stir until heated. Place shrimp and vegetable mixture into a large covered bowl.
6. Return skillet to the heat and add 2 tbsp - oil. Pour eggs into the skillet and scramble until done. Remove eggs to the bowl with shrimp and vegetables.
7. Return skillet to heat and add 1 tbsp oil. Add rice and stir to heat and coat with oil.
8. Season rice with salt and pepper and let rice sit in skillet without stirring for about 2 minutes.
9. Stir rice and add the shrimp, vegetables and eggs. Serve hot.

Nutritional Facts: based on a 1 cup serving

Calories - 421   Sodium - 271mg
Protein - 16g   Potassium - 285mg
Carbohydrates - 53g   Phosphorus - 218mg
Fat - 16g   Calcium - 71mg
Cholesterol - 244mg   Fiber - 2.5g

Chicken - another good source of protein, and a very affordable poultry. Check out some of my homemade recipes:

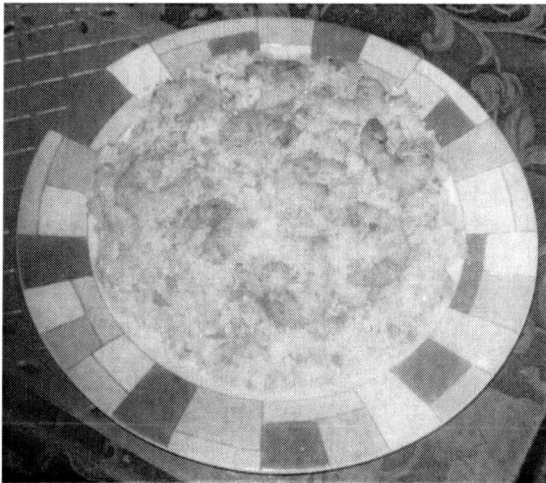

CHICKEN AND VEGETABLE CACCIATORA

Ingredients:

1 lb - whole wheat penne pasta
2 tbsp - olive oil
2 boneless, skinless
Chicken breast halves,
Cut into strips
½ large bell pepper, cut
Into strips
½ med. Onion, thinly sliced
1 tsp - Mrs. Dash (table blend)
1 tbsp - garlic powder
1 tsp - worchestire sauce

1 tbsp - dried parsley
2 tsp - dried basil
½ cup - water
1 cup - fat free chicken broth
2 fresh plum tomatoes cut,
into pieces
Grated Parmesan cheese,
(optional)
1 tsp - season salt
1 tbsp - onion powder
½ tsp - red wine vinegar

Instructions:

Cook pasta - follow packaged direction. Drain and set aside. Meanwhile, heat oil in a large pot or Dutch oven over medium heat. Season chicken with Mrs. Dash, garlic powder, onion powder, and season salt. Add chicken to the pot, and brown both sides. Remove the chicken and transfer to a platter of some sort, and set aside.

Place bell pepper, onion, garlic, tomatoes, parsley, basil, broth and water in pot, stir to blend together and simmer for 10 minutes.

Add chicken, fresh tomatoes and cooked pasta, stir just until heated. Top with grated parmesan cheese (if desired).

Nutritional Facts: based on a ½ cup serving

Calories- 200
Fat - 5g
Sat Fat - 2g
Cholesterol - 25mg
Sodium - 260mg

Fiber - 8g
Protein - 20g
Carbohydrates - 40g
Potassium - 260mg

LEMON SMOTHERED CHICKEN LEGS

Ingredients:

6 chicken legs
1 ½ cups - flour
1 brown paper bag or plastic Ziploc bag

Dry seasonings: 1 tsp - season salt, 1 tbsp - Mrs. Dash (table blend), 1 tbsp - garlic powder, 1 tbsp - onion powder, 1 tsp - black pepper, ½ tsp - creole seasoning.

1 tsp - worchestire sauce	olive oil - to coat bottom of a skillet
Zest and juice of one lemon	½ cup - red pepper - chopped
1 tsp - red wine vinegar	1 cup - green onion - chopped
1 ½ cup - chicken broth	½ tsp - minced ginger
1 cup - water	½ cup - shallots - chopped
1 onion - chopped	1 garlic clove - chopped
1 bell pepper - chopped	dash of hot sauce (optional)

Combine season salt, Mrs. Dash, garlic powder, onion powder, black pepper and creole seasoning, and season chicken with the dry seasoning mixture. Place flour in bag, and coat two chicken legs at a time, and shake off the excess, and repeat until all chicken as been evenly coated. In a deep skillet, drizzle oil to coat the bottom of the skillet with and combine oil with 1 tbsp - margarine.

On medium high heat, brown the chicken on all sides. Then add water, broth, wine vinegar, worchestire sauce, zest hot sauce and juice of one lemon. Then add the onion, bell pepper, red pepper, green onions, shallots and garlic. Bring to a boil, and simmer on medium heat for 1 hour.

Note: check back at the nutritional facts, for chicken parts of protein intake

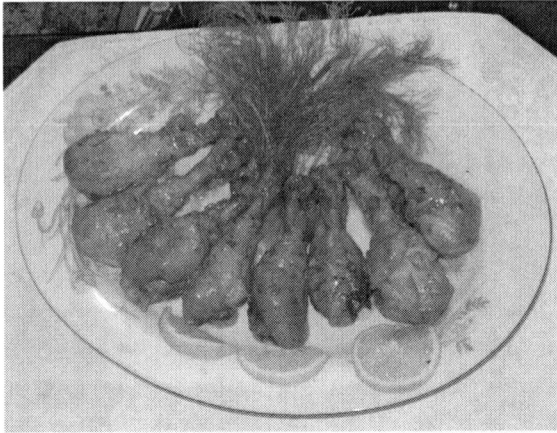

KICKIN CHICKEN FAJITAS

Ingredients:

3 tbsp - canola oil, divided
2 cup - green pepper strips
2 cup - sliced onions
1 lb - chicken breast strips
1 tsp - chili powder
½ tsp - cumin
½ tsp - cinnamon

lime juice
8 small flour tortillas
2 cup - shredded lettuce
1 ½ cup - shredded mozzarello
1 ½ cup - guacamole
½ cup - salsa
1 cup - sour cream

Instructions:

Heat 2 tbsp - oil in a large skillet over medium-high heat. Add bell pepper and onion; cook and stir 5 minutes or until crisp-tender. Remove from skillet, set aside.

Add remaining 1 tbsp - oil to skillet, add chicken, chili powder, cumin and cinnamon. Stir to coat well. Cook 3 minutes or chicken is no longer pink. Sprinkle with lime juice to taste.

Warm tortillas according to package directions. To assemble fajitas, spoon chicken and vegetables down the center of each tortilla; top with lettuce, cheese, guacamole, salsa and sour cream. Fold the bottom of each tortilla up over the filling, and fold in the sides to overlap. Serve immediately.

Nutritional Facts:

Calories - 300
Fat - 15g
Sat Fat - 6g
Cholesterol - 60mg
Sodium - 490mg
Potassium - 240mg
Chicken - white - 3 oz serving - 185mg of phosphorus

Carbohydrates - 21g
Fiber - 1g
Sugar - 3g
Protein - 30g
Omega - 3 - 0g

Glo's tip: I make these fajitas as a snack and also dinner at times, you can also substitute the chicken for shrimp

SIMPLE ROASTED CHICKEN

Ingredients:

1 (3 ½ to 4 lb) - whole chicken
4 tbsp - tub margarine
½ tsp - dry thyme
½ tsp - season salt
1 tbsp - Mrs. Dash (herb and garlic)
Seasoning

1 lemon, peel finely grated
1 small onion, chopped
2 celery stalks, chopped
½ tsp - black pepper
1 tbsp - garlic powder
1 tbsp - onion powder

Instructions:

Preheat oven to 375 degrees. Rinse chicken and pat dry with paper towels. Season chicken inside and out with season salt, Mrs. Dash, black pepper, garlic powder, and onion powder; set aside.

Place margarine in a small bowl. Add thyme and lemon peel; stir to combine. Gently loosen the skin (but don't remove) - the skin of the chicken breast. Forming a pocket between the skin and meat. Carefully spread the margarine mixture on meat under the skin; replace skin. Cut lemon in half and squeeze lemon juice over the entire chicken.

Place lemon halves, onion and celery in chicken cavity. Tie the legs together with kitchen twine. Place chicken on the rack in a roasting pan, or a baking dish. Roast for 1 hour. Remove from oven and let stand loosely covered with foil 5 minutes before carving.

Nutritional Facts: based on 3 oz - serving

Calories - 635   Carbohydrates - 2g   Protein - 58g
Fiber - 0g   Fat - 43g   Sat Fat - 16g
Cholesterol - 210mg   Sodium - 175mg
Phosphorus - dark - 154mg white - 185mg

CHICKEN & PASTA DISH

Ingredients: This is a one dish meal

3 cup - cooked pasta (of your choice)
8 oz - chicken breast, cut into strips
2 garlic cloves, chopped
¼ cup - early virgin olive oil (EVOO)
1 ½ cup - broccoli florets, chopped
½ cup - green onions, chopped
1 cup - red peppers, chopped
1 tsp - ground basil
¼ tsp -cayenne pepper
¾ cup - white wine
1 cup - low sodium chicken broth

Instructions:

In a large skillet, saute garlic. Add chicken breast strips and brown. Add remaining ingredients and simmer for 15 minutes. Toss with cooked pasta and serve immediately.

Nutritional Facts: based on one (1) cup serving

Protein - 19g
Sodium - 169mg
Fat - 16g
Potassium - 411mg
Carbohydrates - 26g
Calcium - 75mg
Calories - 335
Phosphorus - 196mg

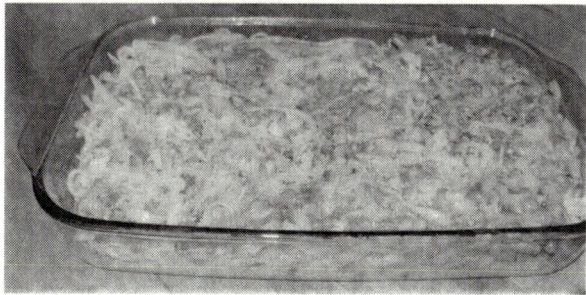

TURKEY SALAD WITH BALSAMIC VINGERETTE

Ingredients:

6 cups - shredded iceberg lettuce
3 cups - chopped turkey breast - pre boiled
1/3 lb - thinly sliced prosciutto, chopped
½ lb - shredded mozarello cheese
1 can (15 ounces) - garbanzo beans, drained, and rinsed
6 medium plum tomatoes, chopped
1 cup - pitted ripe olives, sliced
8 green onions, thinly sliced (½ cup)
½ cup chopped fresh basil

Instructions for Salad:

Combine lettuce, turkey, proscuitto, cheese, beans, tomatoes, olives, onions and basil in large bowl.

Dressing:

2 cloves garlic, minced
1 tbsp Dijon mustard
3 tbsp balsamic vinegar
2/3 cup olive oil
1 tbsp dried Italian seasoning
¼ tsp salt

Instructions for Dressing:

Combine garlic, mustard and vinegar in small bowl. Gradually add oil, beating with wire whisk until well blended. Stir in Italian seasoning, salt and pepper. Sprinkle shredded cheese on top. Add ½ cup dressing.

Toss to coat. If you desire a moister salad, add more dressing.

Nutritional Facts:

Turkey - based on a 1 oz serving - Turkey Breast

Protein - 9g	Sodium - 23mg	Potassium - 117mg
Calories - 50	Phosphorus - 114mg	

Mozzarella cheese - 1 oz - 105mg - phosphorus

Tomato - cooked from fresh - ½ cup serving

Protein - 2g	Sodium - 13mg	Potassium - 312mg
Calories - 30	Phosphorus - 35mg	

Tomato - canned - cooked - ½ cup serving

Protein - 1g	Sodium - 195mg	Potassium - 265mg
Calories - 24	Phosphorus - 23mg	

Note: Garbanzo beans - run in the high category of phosphorus, so be careful with your phosphorus intake

TURKEY MEAT LOAF

Ingredients:

1 lb lean ground turkey
1 large egg, whole
½ cup - low-sodium ketchup
1 cup - bell pepper, chopped
1 tbsp - onion powder
1 cup - celery, chopped

½ cup - plain breadcrumbs
1 cup - onions, chopped
½ tsp - worchestire sauce
1 tbsp - garlic powder
½ tsp - season salt

Instructions:

Preheat oven to 350 degrees. Combine all ingredients, and mix well. Bake in a loaf pan at 350 degrees for 25 minutes.

Nutritional Facts:

Calories - 226.53
Protein - 20g
Carbohydrates - 14.52g
Fiber - 1.90g
Fat - 9.61g
Omega - 3 - .10g
Omega - 6 - 1.86g
Phosphorus - 249.92mg
Potassium - 298.64mg
Sodium - 102.20mg

Pork - referred to as the other white meat - Pork is very affordable, and a another great source of protein, but the phosphorus intake runs in the highest category. Check out some of my real easy to prepare and cook, pork recipes below:

PEPPERED PORK TENDERLOIN

Ingredient:

1 tbsp - black pepper
1 ½ to 2 lb pork tenderloin
½ cup - 1 stick - unsalted butter
1 tsp - season salt

3 tbsp - brandy
¼ cup - heavy cream
1 tsp - Mrs. Dash (table blend)
3 cloves - garlic - minced

Instructions:

Sprinkle pepper on all sides of tenderloin. Gently press pepper into pork. Slice pork into ¼ inch-thick slices. Place a large skillet over medium-high heat. Add ½ stick butter and stir until melted. Add pork to butter and saute for 2 minutes. Turn pork over and saute for an additional 2 minutes. Add garlic to pan and saute for 30 seconds. Reduce heat to low, add brandy and cook for 2 minutes. Add remaining butter to pan and stir until melted. Add cream and heat until warm. Season with season salt, Mrs. Dash, and pepper. Serve sauce over pork slices.

Nutritional Facts: based on 3 oz - serving

Calories - 280
Sodium - 85mg
Protein - 28g
Pork - 3 oz serving -
Sat fat - 4g
Cholesterol - 90mg

Fat - 13g
Carbohydrates - 12
Fiber - 2g
phosphorus - 224mg

SMOTHERED PORK CHOPS

Ingredients:

4 - bone-in pork chops
½ cup - buttermilk, or
½ cup - mocha mix -
  (dialysis patients)
1 egg
½ tsp - creole seasoning
1 tbsp - garlic powder
½ tsp - season salt
1 cup - flour

1 ½ tbsp - olive oil
1 ½ cups - onions - sliced
1 cup - bell pepper - chopped
2 garlic cloves - chopped
2 tbsp - butter (preferably tub margarine)
1 tbsp - onion powder
2 ½ cups - chicken broth (low sodium)
kitchen bouquet
2 tsp - worchestire sauce

Glo's Tip: Being a dialysis patient, it's more sensible to use tub margarine, when the recipe calls for butter and if chicken broth is a part of the recipe - I use low sodium chicken broth - so that I can control the sodium in the recipe. **Remember dialysis patient are supposed to eat no more than 2000 milligrams of sodium a day.**

Instructions:

Season chops in creole seasoning, garlic & onion powder. Place flour and season salt in a bowl, and whisk together. Place the egg and milk in another bowl and mix well. Dip the chops in the egg milk mixture and then coat in the flour. In a deep skillet, on medium-high heat brown the chops on both sides.

Turn the heat to medium-low, and add the broth, then add the onions, bell pepper and garlic to skillet and cover. Let simmer for 1 hour.

Remove the chops and transfer to plate or platter. Meanwhile scrap the bottom of the skillet and in a cup - measure ¾ cup of flour and 2 tbsp - butter, and make into a paste, and add to the skillet and whisk until combined, add broth, worchestire sauce and a dash of kitchen bouquet, whisk until gravy consistency, add chops in the gravy and cook for five minutes.

Nutritional Facts: based on 1 oz serving

Protein - 9g
Potassium - 97mg

Sodium - 21mg
Phosphorus - 92mg

Calories -76

BRAISED BEEF WITH MUSHROOM SAUCE

Ingredients:

1 (2 - 2 ½ lb.) - beef eye round roast
1 tsp - Mrs. Dash (Italian seasoning)
1 cup - onion - finely chopped
½ cup - celery - finely chopped
3 ½ cup - fresh mushrooms, halved, divided

1 tbsp - olive oil
½ tsp - season salt
½ tsp - pepper
1 ½ cup - beef broth

Instructions:

Trim fat from beef. Combine Italian seasoning, season salt, and pepper; rub onto meat. Finely chopped ½ cup - mushrooms.

In a 5-quart dutch oven, brown meat on all sides in hot oil. Add onions, celery and chopped mushrooms. Cook 3 minutes.

Add broth, bring to boil; reduce heat. Simmer covered for 1 ½ hours. Stir in remaining mushrooms, cover and cook for 15 minutes or until meat is tender. Remove roast from pan; cover and keep warm. Bring mushrooms and broth to boil; cook 5 minutes or until slightly thickened.

Thinly slice meat and serve with mushroom sauce over rice or hot cooked noodles - follow package directions for both.

Nutritional Facts - based on 3 oz - serving

Calories - 230
Fat - 13g
Potassium - 510mg

Cholesterol - 60mg
Sat Fat - 4g
Fiber - 1g

Carbohydrates - 4g
Sodium - 355mg
Protein - 24g

Note: phosphorus intake - 3 oz serving - beef eye round - 177mg

CHICKEN FRIED STEAK WITH CREAMY MUSHROOM SAUCE

Ingredients:

1 lb. beef tip steak
2 large egg, beaten
1 cup - flour
1 tbsp - garlic powder
1 cup - Mushrooms - sliced
2 tbsp - tub margarine

½ in. - oil in skillet for frying
1 cup - Planko bread crumbs
½ tsp - season salt
1 tbsp - onion powder
¾ cup - flour

Instructions:

Cut steak into 4 even pieces. Place steak between 2 sheets of plastic wrap. You can use unseasoned meat tenderizer or a small heavy frying pan, pound meat until ½ in. thick. Dry meat with paper towels.

Place eggs in a mixing bowl. Place breadcrumbs and flour in a second bowl. Dip steaks in egg and then coat in breadcrumb flour mixture. Repeat egg and breadcrumb mixture with remaining steaks.

Heat ½ in. of oil in a large skillet. Add steak and cook until coating is golden brown, about 2 to 3 minutes on each side. Remove meat from skillet, and set aside in oven at 300 degrees.

Scrap brown bits from bottom of skillet, then add ¾ cup flour and 2 tbsp - margarine to skillet, and whisk together, until smooth, and then began to add chicken broth, until the right consistency. Add mushroom slices and stir for 2 minutes. Take Steaks out of oven, and serve on platter, with mushroom sauce poured on top.

Nutritional Facts: based on 1 oz serving

Protein - 9g   Sodium - 21mg   Potassium - 97mg
Phosphorus - 69mg   Calories - 63

Note: Mushrooms - ½ cup serving raw - 130mg - potassium
Mushrooms - ½ cup serving, cooked - 278mg - potassium

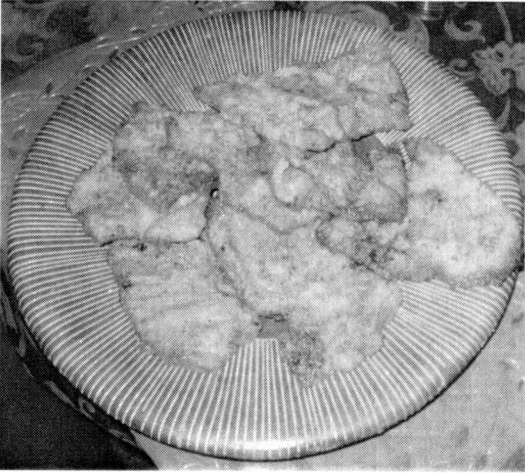

SIMPLE T-BONE GRILLED STEAK

Ingredients:

2 - T-bone beef steaks
4 tsp - olive oil
2 - garlic cloves
½ tsp - Mrs. Dash - table blend seasoning
¼ tsp - worchestire sauce

2 tbsp - fresh basil, chopped
1 tsp - lemon pepper
½ tsp - season salt

Glo's tip: you can use 1 ½ tsp - dried basil, if you prefer

Instructions:

Preheat indoor grill to medium. In small bowl, stir together basil, olive oil, Worchester sauce and garlic. Rub over both sides of steaks. Season steak with Mrs. Dash, lemon pepper, and season salt or black pepper, if you prefer.

Grill directly to desired doneness for about 15 minutes for medium-rare. 14-16 minutes for medium, and 20 minutes for well done. Turning once.

Nutritional Facts: based on 3 oz serving

Calories - 540mg
Fiber - 0g
Sodium - 120mg

Protein - 44g
Fat - 39g
Potassium - 715mg

Carbohydrates - 1g
Cholesterol - 130mg

Note: based on a 1 oz serving - the phosphorus intake in T-bone steak is 69mg

BREADED VEAL CUTLETS

Ingredients:

4 (4 oz) - veal cutlets
1/8 tsp - garlic powder
2 eggs, well beaten
2 tbsp - milk
1 lemon wedges

1 cup - Italian breadcrumbs
canola oil for frying
fresh parsley - finely minced
1 tsp - season salt
Mrs. Dash (garlic and herb)

Instructions:

Season cutlets with garlic powder, season salt, and Mrs. Dash.

Whisk eggs and milk together in a small bowl. Place breadcrumbs in a shallow dish or plate. Dip cutlets into egg mixture, then into breadcrumbs to coat.

Heat ¼ in. of oil in a large skillet over medium heat. Add cutlets, cook cutlets for 2 minutes on both sides or until golden. Remove cutlets to paper towels to drain. Transfer to a warm serving platter, sprinkle with parsley and serve with lemon wedges.

Nutritional Facts: Based on 3 oz serving

Calories - 325
Cholesterol - 180mg
Carbohydrates - 10g
Omega 3 - 0g

Fat - 15g
Sodium - 325mg
Fiber - 1g

Sat Fat - 5g
Potassium - 270mg
Protein - 26g

Note: 1 oz = serving of veal cutlet - contains 82mg of phosphorus

VEAL CUTLETS W/HERB CRUST

Ingredients:

2 (4 oz.) - veal cutlets
½ cup - flour
1 egg, beaten
1 cup - Italian breadcrumbs
1 tbsp - garlic powder
¼ tsp - fresh parsley, chopped

¼ tsp - fresh chives, chopped
1 tbsp - tub margarine
2 tbsp - lemon juice
1 tsp - Mrs. Dash (garlic and herb)
1 tbsp - onion powder
½ tsp - season salt

Instructions:

Place veal between 2 sheets of wax paper. Using the flat side of a meat mallet, pound veal until ¼ in. thick. Remove wax paper.

For coating and dipping effect, a platter or plate for flour, a bowl for beaten egg, and a platter or plate for breadcrumb mixture with parley and chives.

Coat veal with flour, then dip in beaten egg, and finally breadcrumb mixture, and repeat these steps for the remaining veal cutlets.

In large skillet, cook veal in butter over medium for 2 to 3 minutes or until juices run clear, turning once. Remove veal to serving plates. Keep warm.

Stir lemon juice into drippings in skillet. Pour lemon mixture over veal just before serving. Sprinkle with additional chopped chives. If desired.

Nutritional Facts: based on a 3 oz serving

Calories - 400
Fat - 13g
Carbohydrates - 3l7g

Sodium - 263mg
Sat Fat - 2g
Fiber - 1g

Omega - 3 - 0g
Cholesterol - 212mg
Protein - 31g

Note: a 1 oz serving of veal contains 82mg of phosphorus

EASY AND SIMPLE COMFORT AT HOME BEEF STEW

Ingredients:

1 tbsp - olive oil
2 lb beef stewing meat
½ tsp - season salt
2 cloves garlic, minced
1 tbsp - garlic powder
1 tsp - worchestire sauce
1 8 oz - can - tomato sauce

2 tsp - dried thyme
1 bay leaf
½ tsp - black pepper
8 oz mushrooms, sliced
1 tbsp - onion powder
4 stalks - celery, chopped
2 cup - beef or chicken broth

Using a slow cooker or pressure cooker:
Heat olive oil in a large skillet over medium-high heat. Season beef with season salt, garlic powder, onion powder and pepper. Brown in olive oil in small batches. When beef is browned, put into slow cooker. Add the rest of the ingredients. Stir to combine. Cook on high 4 hours, or on low for 8 hours, whichever is your preference. Discard bay leaf before serving.

For Pressure Cooker method:
Season beef with season salt and pepper. Place the pan of the pressure cooker (at least 6 quarts) on medium-high heat. Add the olive oil and ¼ of the beef. Brown the beef, then remove from pan and set aside, while you brown the other batches of beef. Once all the beef is browned, place all of it back into the pan. Add the remaining ingredients and stir to combine. Lock pressure lid into place. Bring to pressure over high heat. Lower heat and cook for 20 minutes. Release pressure slowly. Discard bay leaf. Season with season salt, garlic powder, onion powder and pepper before serving.

Nutritional Facts: based on a ½ cup serving

Calories - 319
Protein - 31.51g
Cholesterol - 94.5mg

Sodium - 681mg
Potassium - 429mg
Fat - 13.57g

Fiber - 3.0g
Carb - 16.93g
Omega - 3 - 0g

Note: 1 oz serving - beef stew meat - contains 69mg of phosphorus

LAMB SKEWERS W/ DILLED LEMON SAUCE

Ingredients:

Boneless top round lamb, cut into 1-inch cubes (about 24 ct.)
6 large - white mushrooms, cut into quarters
1 large - red bell pepper, cored, seeded and cut into 1-inch pieces (about 24 ct.)
A dozen cherry tomatoes, halved and seeded
¼ cup - fresh parsley - parsley chopped

For marinade:

Ingredients:

6 tbsp - dry red wine
4 tbsp - soy sauce
1 tbsp - garlic - finely minced
2 tbsp - fresh parsley - chopped

:

Dilled Lemon Sauce:

Ingredients:

1 cup - plain nonfat yogurt, drained
1 tbsp - fresh lemon juice
1 tsp - finely grated lemon zest
¼ cup - extra virgin olive oil
¼ tsp - ground black pepper
1 tbsp - garlic & onion powder
1 tsp - season salt
2 tsp - fresh dill - chopped

To sprinkle on the lamb after it marinades:

1 tsp - black pepper   1 tbsp - garlic powder
1 tbsp - onion powder   1 tsp - Mrs. Dash (table blend seasoning)
½ tsp - season salt

Instructions:
Combine the yogurt, lemon juice and zest in a small bowl. Slowly drizzle in the olive oil, whisking constantly until smooth and slightly thick.

Instructions:

1. Combine all the ingredients for the marinade in a bowl. Add the lamb and the mushrooms; toss to coat. Set aside at room temperature for 1 hour. Meanwhile soak about 24 bamboo skewers (about 6 inches long) in water for 1 hour.

2. Preheat the oven to 450 F. Lightly grease a baking sheet.
3. Thread each of the skewers with one piece each of red pepper, lamb, a mushroom quarter and a tomato half.
4. Arrange skewers on the prepared baking sheet and bake for 5 minutes, until it sizzles. Immediately after baking, sprinkle the skewers well with the chopped parsley. Serve immediately with the Dilled Lemon Sauce.

Nutritional Facts: based on 3 oz serving

Lamb kabobs, loin and lean - has about 190mg of phosphorus, which runs in the higher category of phosphorus intake

Protein - 25.5g of protein - a great source of protein, which runs in the highest category of protein intake

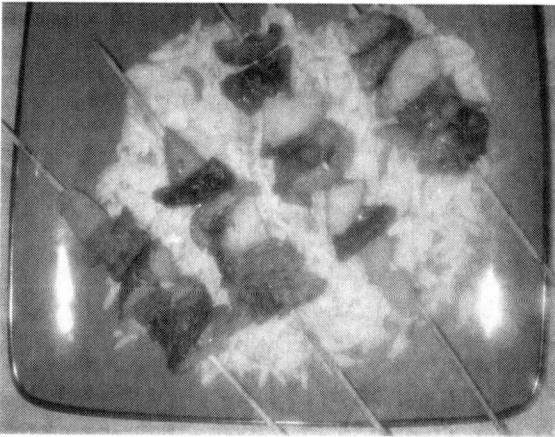

TOFU:

PASTA PRIMAVERA SALAD W/TOFU:

Ingredients:

8 oz. Uncooked bow rotini pasta

2 cup - broccoli florets

½ (16 oz.) - container of firm tofu, Drained and cut into ½ inch cubes

1 can artichoke hearts, drained and Quartered

1 (8 oz.) bottle reduced fat Italian salad dressing

1 small red bell pepper chopped

1 shallot chopped

1 tbsp onion powder

1 tbsp garlic powder

pinch salt

pinch pepper

Note: You can make the garlic and herb salad dressing from my list of salad dressing recipes (that start on page . . . .) Or you can try ready made Italian salad dressing in a bottle.

Instructions:

Cook pasta according to package directions. Drain and rinse with cold water.

In a large bowl, combine pasta, broccoli, tofu, artichokes, bell pepper, shallot, salt, pepper, onion powder, garlic powder, and dressing. Toss to coat. Cover and chill for an hour and serve at room temperature.

Facts:

Tofu (if you haven't tried it) it's a custard-like food made from soybeans and is a great source of protein. It's usually sold in the refrigerator section of the produce department. When you open it at home, you should keep it in a sealed container in the refrigerator. Water should be added to the container to keep the tofu from drying out. The water should be changed daily.

(If you are a vegetarian, it's an affordable meat substitute for your recipe. Also great in a meatless stir-fry recipe. Remember it's an already cooked food, so all you have to do is heat it up).

NOTE: A soy burger is equivalent to two or three ounces of protein

Nutrition Facts:

Calories - 71, carbohydrates - 7g, protein - 3g, fat - 4g, fiber - 1g, cholesterol - 2mg, sodium - 160mg

Vegetables

The vegetables are low biological protein, check back at the chapter on Albumin - for biological protein in foods.

Now, let's talk about potatoes first. It is a fact that potatoes and most potato dishes are very high in potassium, so if you are on a potassium restricted diet and plan to eat yams, potatoes, or sweet potatoes once in awhile, leeching should be included in the preparation of these vegetables. *Leeching* is a process that will pull out or soak part of the potassium from the potatoes, sweet potatoes, and yams. You can never remove all the potassium only part of it, so remember to take those binders.

To Dialyze Potatoes, you need to follow these steps:

1. Peel the skin off
2. Cut the potato into small pieces such as: cubes, round slices (that could be later, put back together, wrap in foil and bake it - for a bake potato recipe), you can also cut potato lengthwise in strips (these can be French fries)
3. Soak them in water for at least four hours or overnight in the refrigerator
4. Throw away the soaking water
5. Cook the potato in fresh water in the oven or fry them

I would like to share some of my easy to prepare and cook potato recipes: on the following page - "POTATO, POTATO"

An Assortment Of Recipes Made With Potatoes

Roasted Garlic Mashed Potatoes

Southern Style Potato Salad

Yukon Gold Mashed Potatoes
With Chives

Vegetable Sides:

Broccoli and Cauliflower
Au Gratin
Savory Butternut Squash Crisp
Brussel Sprouts with Potatoes
Bok Choy
Rice Pilaf w/Parsley
Stuffed Peppers
Sugar Snap Peas
Roasted Asparagus
Baked Beets
Glazed Minted Orange Carrots

"POTATO, POTATO"

ROASTED GARLIC MASHED POTATOES

Ingredients:

4 large red potatoes
(peeled and cut into 2
Inch pieces)
2 tbsp - roasted garlic clove
½ tsp - black pepper
1 ½ tbsp - sour cream

1 tsp - salt
2-3 tsp - warm low fat milk
2 tbsp - extra virgin olive oil
2 tbsp - tub margarine

Instructions:

Put the potatoes in a medium saucepan and add just enough cold water to cover the potatoes. Add 1 tsp salt and bring to a simmer over medium heat. Do not boil. Cook for 12 to 15 minutes or until the potato are just tender enough to slide off a paring knife when pierced. Drain well and return to the pan.

Mash potatoes w/cream, margarine, olive oil, warm milk, pepper, sour cream, and sour cream, mix all ingredients well in the mashed potatoes. Add more salt to taste

Nutritional Facts: based on ½ cup serving

Calories - 81
Potassium - 314mg

Protein - 2g
Phosphorus - 50mg

Sodium - 318mg

SOUTHERN STYLE POTATO SALAD

Ingredients:

5 large red potatoes
½ cup - mayonnaise
2 tsp - yellow mustard
2 tbsp - pickle relish
2 boiled eggs
½ tsp - sugar
½ tsp - ranch dressing
Paprika - to garnish on top

1 tsp - salt
1 tbsp - garlic powder
1 tbsp - onion powder
½ cup - onion, chopped
½ cup - bell pepper
1 ½ cup - red pepper
1 cup - celery, chopped

In a saucepan, place potatoes in cold water, enough to cover them. Bring to a boil for 8 to 10 minutes.

Drain well, and place in a serving bowl. Add mayonnaise, mustard, ranch dressing, sugar, relish, salt, garlic powder, onion powder, onions, bell pepper, red pepper, celery, and mix well, then crumble the eggs in the potato mixture. Garnish with paprika on top.

Nutritional Facts: based on a ½ cup serving

Calories - 179
Protein - 3.5g
Sodium - 661mg
Potassium - 317mg
Phosphorus - 65mg

YUKON GOLD MASHED POTATOES WITH CHIVES

Ingredients:

1 ½ lb. Peeled Yukon gold potatoes
Cut into 1 in. cubes
2 cloves garlic - chopped
2 cups low sodium chicken broth
¾ cup - butter milk or mocha mix (to watch phosphorus intake)
1 tbsp - minced fresh chives or green onions
1 tsp - creole seasoning
1 tbsp - garlic & onion powder
¼ tsp - pepper
¼ tsp - salt
1 ½ tbsp - margarine (tub - for dialysis pts.)

Instructions:

In a saucepan, combine the potatoes, garlic and broth. Cover and bring to a boil over high heat. Reduce the heat to medium-low and simmer until are potatoes are tender. 10-12 minutes.

Drain the potatoes in a colander. Then return the potatoes to the same saucepan. Add the milk. With a potato masher or handheld mixer, mash the potatoes until they become fluffy and light. Mix in the buttermilk, creole seasoning, garlic & onion powder, pepper, salt and margarine. Stir in the chives or green onion. Serve immediately.

Nutritional Facts: based on a ½ cup serving

Sodium - 42 mg
Protein - 4 g
Cholesterol - 2 mg
Carbohydrates - 20 g
Carbohydrates - 20 g
Fiber - 3 g
Saturated Fat - 1 g
phosphorus - 50mg

BROCCOLI AND CAULIFLOWER AU GRATIN

Ingredients:

1 (16 oz) pkg of fresh broccoli and cauliflower florets
½ cup - reduced fat mayonnaise
½ cup - shredded mozzarella cheese
½ cup - shredded parmesan cheese
3 green onions, sliced
1 garlic clove, minced
1 tbsp - Dijon mustard
1/8 tsp - ground red pepper or cayenne pepper
2 tbsp - Italian seasoned breadcrumbs
¼ tsp - paprika

Instructions:

Preheat oven to 350 degrees. Arrange florets in a microwave steamer, for about 5 minutes or boil in water for about 6 to 8 minutes or until crisp-tender. Drain well.

Lightly grease 2-quart baking dish. Arrange florets in baking pan.

Stir together mayonnaise. Mozzarella cheese, parmesan cheese, green onions, garlic, mustard and red pepper. Spoon over florets. Sprinkle with breadcrumbs and paprika.

Bake for 20 to 25 minutes or until golden.

Nutritional Facts: based on a ½ cup serving

Calories - 140
Fat - 8g
Sat Fat - 3g
Cholesterol - 20mg
Sodium - 500mg
Potassium - 210mg
Carbohydrates - 9g

Fiber - 3g
Protein - 7g
Omega - 3 - 0g

SAVORY BUTTERNUT SQUASH CRISP

Ingredients:

1 (2 lb.) - Butternut squash, peeled, seeded and cut into ¾ inch. Cubes
½ cup - tub margarine. divided
1 tsp - salt, divided
¼ tsp - black pepper
1 cup - onions, chopped
2 cup - Italian breadcrumbs
¼ tsp - crush dried rosemary
¼ cup - walnuts, chopped (optional)

Instructions:

Preheat oven to 400 degrees. Bring large pot of water to a boil. Drop in squash cubes, cook 7-8 minutes or until fork tender. Drain well. Spoon squash into 3-quart baking dish. Toss with 1 tbsp - of the margarine. ¼ tsp - salt and pepper. Set aside.

Meanwhile, melt remaining 3 tbsp - margarine in large skillet over medium heat. Add onion, saute' 5 minutes or until tender. Stir in bread cubes, remaining ¼ tsp salt and rosemary; saute' 1 to 2 minutes to coat with margarine. Stir in walnuts, spoon over squash.

Bake 10 minutes or until bread cubes are lightly browned, tossing before serving.

Nutritional Facts: based on ½ cup serving

Calories - 260
Fat - 12g
Sat Fat - 7g
Cholesterol - 30mg
Sodium - 425mg

Potassium - 7440mg - yes, it is way too much potassium for a renal diet, just know your limits on potassium intake. Don't over indulge, O.K. This is a very great tasting dish, but what can I say, the potassium is in question.

Carbohydrates - 36g
Fiber - 5g   Note: ½ cup serving of butternut squash
Protein - 4g   has 448mg of potassium
Omega - 3 - 0g

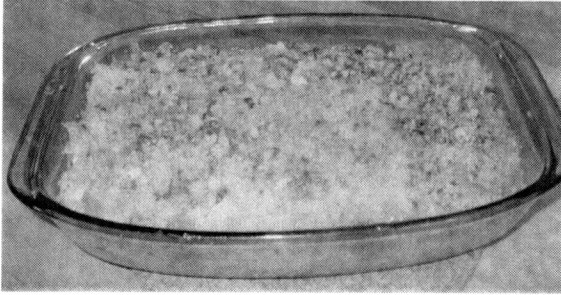

BRUSSEL SPROUTS W/POTATOES:

Ingredients:

1 lb. Brussel Sprouts, fresh
1 large potato, cut in small cubes
1 tbsp butter or margarine
1 onion, chopped
1 bay leaf
1 red bell pepper, cut in chunks

½ cup chicken stock
½ tsp ground black pepper
½ tsp creole seasoning
tbsp garlic powder
1 tbsp onion powder
2 tbsp fresh parsley
cup green onions, chopped

Instructions:

In a large skillet, melt butter over medium heat; cook onion, potato and bay leaf, stirring often, until onion is softened.

If Brussel sprouts are large, cut them in half. Add sprouts, red pepper, and stock; cover and cook for 8 to 10 minutes (add water if necessary).

Season with pepper, Creole seasoning, garlic powder, and onion powder. Sprinkle with parsley and green onions

Nutrition Facts:

Calories - 85, carbohydrates - 50g, protein - 4g, cholesterol - 0mg, sodium - 65mg, fiber - 5g, fat - 2g

Note: ½ cup serving of brussel sprouts, contain 246 mg of potassium, when cooked from raw

BOK CHOY
(try making this dish, it's a change from the usual cabbage with rice dish)

Ingredients:

Buoy Choy
1 cup - sliced yellow onions
2 cups - green onions (chopped)
½ cup - roasted red pepper (they come in a jar - already roasted) - like strips (just dice them up) or fresh red pepper (roasted) - diced
1 tbsp - olive oil
2 tsp - butter
½ tbsp - Creole seasoning
1 tbsp Garlic powder
1 tbsp Onion powder
2 clove garlic, minced
1 tsp. - worchestire sauce
1 lbs. - procuitto - (Italian bacon) or turkey bacon (if you prefer)
Long grain rice - (follow box directions)

Instructions:

Saute the yellow onions, green onions, roasted red peppers in the olive oil & butter (until they are caramelized), then add the cabbage to be saute until wilted over medium heat

Then add the seasonings including the worchestire sauce. Add the procuitto to the cabbage mixture, simmer for about 20 mins. On low heat. Serve hot over rice.

Nutritional Facts: based on a ½ cup serving

Protein - 0.5g
Sodium - 23mg
Potassium - 88mg
Phosphorus - 13mg
Calories - 5

RICE PILAF W/BARLEY

Ingredients:

1 tbsp - margarine
1 small - onion (chopped)
1/3 cup - barley
1/3 cup - white rice
2 cups - low sodium chicken broth
1 carrot - peeled and finely chopped
1 stalk celery - finely chopped
½ tsp - dried thyme
1/8 tsp - ground black pepper

Instructions:

In a medium saucepan, melt margarine over moderate heat. Add onion and cook for about 5 minutes or until soft. Add barley and rice and cook, stirring for 1 minute. Add remaining ingredients and bring to boil. Reduce heat and simmer and cover for 20 minutes or until the liquid is absorbed.

Nutritional Facts: based on a ½ cup serving

Calories - 171, Carbohydrates - 30g, protein - 4g, Fat - 4g, Sodium - 83mg, potassium - 186mg, phosphorus - 80mg

STUFFED PEPPERS

Ingredients:

4 - Green peppers
1 tsp - worchestire sauce
1 tsp - onion powder
1 tsp - garlic powder
½ tsp - ground thyme
1 tbsp - parsley flakes
1 ½ cups - water or chicken broth
½ lb - ground turkey
1 ½ cup - cooked orzo -
    follow package directions

1 medium - onion - finely chopped
1 tsp - creole seasoning
1 medium - celery stalk - finely chopped
1 medium - carrot - shredded
2 clove - garlic - minced
½ cup - shallot - chopped
2 tbsp - apple cider vinegar
3 cups - Italian bread crumbs -
    (for topping)

Instructions:

In a 12-inch skillet over medium heat, brown ground turkey, add celery, carrot, onion, and garlic and cook until tender stirring occasionally, about 10 minutes.

Drain the ground turkey and vegetable mixture from the heat, place in a bowl and mix in vinegar, garlic powder, onion powder, parsley flakes, creole seasonings, and thyme, add the orzo to the meat and vegetable mixture and mix well. Place about 3 tbsp of the mixture in each of the peppers. Sprinkle each pepper with Italian bread crumbs and drizzle with EVOO on top for browning. Pour 1 ½ cup broth to coat the bottom of the baking dish.

Pre-heat oven to 350 degrees and place peppers in the baking dish and bake for 10 to 15 minutes, or until bread crumbs are golden brown.

FYI: There's about 530 mg of potassium in this recipe. Please Dialysis patients watch the potassium intake. (if you need to cut down on potassium in your diet)

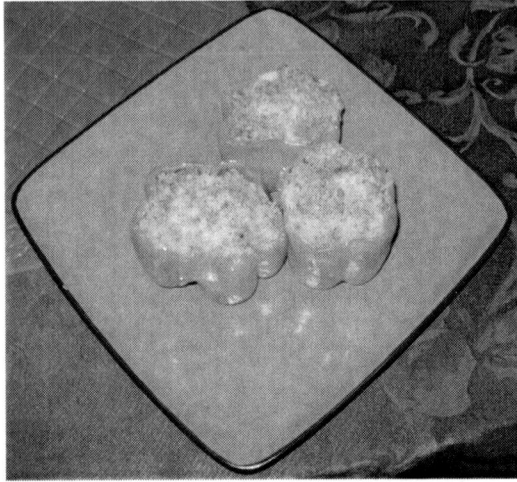

SUGAR SNAP PEAS

Ingredients:

1 lb. Sugar snap peas
1 ½ tbsp butter or margarine
¾ tsp lemon zest or 2 tbsp fresh mint, chopped
Salt and pepper to taste

Instructions:

Add sugar snap peas to a large pot of boiling water, and cook for one minute. Drain and place them into a bowl of ice water to stop the cooking process.

Over medium-low heat, melt butter in a skillet large enough to hold the sugar snap peas. Add the lemon zest or the chopped fresh mint.

Put sugar snap peas in the skillet and toss with butter seasoning mixture. Gently heat sugar snap peas for two minutes or until peas are hot. Serve immediately.

Glo's Tip: Sugar snap peas are also great in vingerette salads; such as my radicchio salad recipe.

Nutritional Facts:

Calories - 81, carbohydrates - 7g, protein - 3.5g, cholesterol - 12g, sodium - 33mg, fiber - 3g, fat - 5g

ROASTED ASPARAGUS

Ingredients:

1 (thin, asparagus spears, 10-12 stalks)
1 cup - fresh basil - finely chopped
1 cup - grated parmesan cheese

2 tbsp - extra virgin olive oil
3 clove garlic

1 tbsp - rice wine vinegar
1 tsp - creole seasoning
1 tbsp - Mrs. Dash (garlic & herb) seasoning
1 tbsp - garlic powder
1 tbsp - onion powder

Instructions:

Preheat oven to 450 F.

Clean asparagus well. Snap one of the spears, and where it snaps, cut the remainder spears at that point.

In a bowl, mix the basil, parmesan cheese, creole seasoning, Mrs. Dash, garlic & onion powder together.

Meanwhile, in a sauce pan, with olive oil, drop the cloves in to be infused in the oil, for about 8 to 10 minutes. Then strain the oil, and mix in the bowl with the basil and dry seasoning mix very thoroughly, then add the rice wine vinegar.

With a brush, vigorously brush the mixture over the asparagus, and then arrange the stalks on a roasting pan and place in oven at 450 F for about 10 to 15 minutes.

Glo's Tip: You can use this same mixture, to prepare artichoke instead. Just steam the artichoke hearts for 2 to 4 minutes. Remove from steamer. Let them sit for a few minutes, then cut in half and drizzle with the infused basil parmesan oil mixture.

Nutritional Facts: (based on a ½ cup - serving)

Calories - 209, carbohydrates - 38g, protein - 6g, cholesterol - 0mg, sodium - 164mg, fiber - 3g, fat - 4g,

FYI: If you are not suppose to get too much potassium in your renal diet, I suggest you cook with the frozen asparagus, because the frozen asparagus will have about 196mg of potassium, and if you are in need of some more potassium in your diet, and yes in some cases a dialysis patient may need to build the potassium in their body, cook with the raw asparagus, because it will give you about 279mg of potassium.

Glo's Tip: A real easy way to cook asparagus - After cleaning and snapping off the spears, season the asparagus with creole seasoning, garlic and onion powder and drizzle with balsamic vinegar and place on a baking pan and bake on 350 degrees for 8 to 10 minutes.

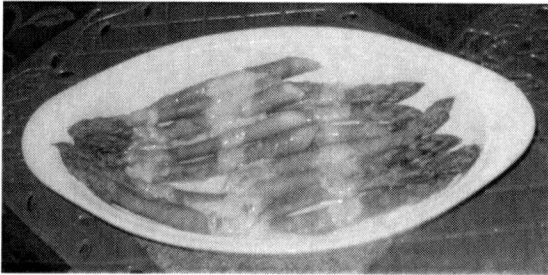

BAKED BEETS

Ingredients:

8 medium beets
1 tbsp - olive oil
1 ½ tsp - red wine vinegar
Zest of 1 orange
1 (8oz.) carton nonfat sour cream
Season all - to taste
Garlic & onion powder - to taste

Instructions:

Preheat oven to 400 F. Place washed and trimmed beets on a sheet of aluminum foil. Fold and seal the foil tightly. Place on baking sheet.

Bake for 1 ½ to 2 hours. Test the beets with a knife, they should be tender but firm.

Cool slightly and peel. Slice the each beet into ¼ inch rounds and place in a bowl. Blend the oil And vinegar and pour over beets. Toss and Season with season oil to taste, garlic & onion Powder to taste. And place in a bowl. Blend the oil and vinegar Arrange the beet slices on a plate or platter. Use a vegetable peeler to remove the zest from the orange. Chop zest finely and stir into the sour cream. Place a dollop of the mixture on top of each beet slice.

Nutritional Facts: (per ½ cup serving)

Calories - 170, carbohydrates - 29g, protein - 6g, fat - 4g, fiber - 6g, cholesterol - 5mg, sodium - 208mg

For the beets - the potassium - is 265mg - for ½ cup serving - sliced

GLAZED MINTED ORANGE CARROTS

Ingredients:

2 lb. Baby carrots, peeled
3 tbsp - butter or margarine
¼ cup - Grand Marnier liqueur or
orange juice
2 tbsp - fresh mint leaves, rinsed & chopped

Instructions:

Cook baby carrots in boiling water until barely tender. Drain and return to pot. Add butter and cook over medium heat until melted. Add liqueur or orange juice. Cook for a couple of minutes more. Stir in mint. Remove from heat and serve.

Nutritional Facts:

A ½ cup of orange juice - is equivalent to 248mg of potassium

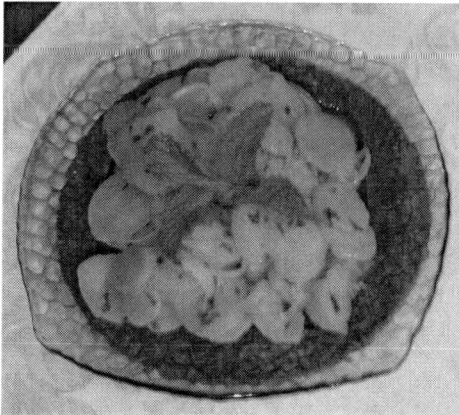

SALADS - I love salads, and I try to have a salad, as a side dish, with maybe whatever meat I chose for lunch, or a sandwich of some sort. Being fortunate to have a great farmers market, right in my backyard in wine country (Napa), I can purchase some of the best and freshest vegetables and fruits at my neighborhood farmers market, Larry's Produce. I would like to share some of my favorite summer salads, that I prepare very often. I even have some recipes to share for fruit and vegetable salsa, slaw and recipes for added garnishes for various meat and seafood dishes.

SALAD CHOICES

Radicchio Salad
Autumn Pear Salad
With Glazed Pecans
Fennel Celery Salad
Grapefruit and Avocado Salad
Cool Sweet & Spicy Cucumber Salad
Tropical Fruit w/Cool Fruit Vinegar Dressing
Kumquat Salad
Watercress Orzo Salad
Renal friendly Chef Salad

RADICCHIO SALAD

Ingredients:

½ lb. Radicchio, shredded - (2 cups)
1 medium onion, thinly sliced
½ cup red wine
1 tart apple, cored and cut in small cubes

Instructions:

Place radicchio, onion, red wine, and apples in a pot. Bring to a boil. Cover and simmer over low heat, for 20 minutes or until all ingredients are tender crisp.

Nutritional Facts: based on a ½ cup serving

Calories - 65   Carbohydrates - 11g
Protein - 1g   Cholesterol - 0mg
Sodium - 16mg   Fiber - 3g
Fat - 0g

AUTUMN PEAR SALAD
WITH GLAZED PEACANS

Ingredients:

1 egg white, beaten
2 tbsp - maple syrup
2 tsp - dark brown sugar
¼ tsp - salt
1 ½ cups - pecan halves,
Roasted

2 small ripe pears, thinly sliced
6 cups - mixed baby greens
½ to 2/3 cup light raspberry vinaigrette
or red wine vinaigrette dressing
fresh raspberries (optional)

Instructions:

Calories - 280
Sat Fat - 2g
Sodium - 290mg
Carbohydrates - 23g
Sugars - 14g
Omega - 3 - 0g

Fat - 21g
Cholesterol - 0mg
Potassium - 165mg
Fiber - 4g
Protein - 4g

Note: a 2 oz serving of roasted pecans - contains 170mg of phosphorus

FENNEL CELERY SALAD

Ingredients

2 fennel bulbs, thinly sliced
2 stalks of celery hearts, thinly sliced
2 tbsp red wine vinegar
2 tsp extra virgin olive oil
Salt & pepper to taste
Garlic and onion powder to taste

Instructions:

In a bowl, cut fennel bulbs and celery hearts into thin slices. Add red wine vinegar, olive oil, salt, pepper, garlic and onion powder and Mix all together and Serve.

Glo's Tip: Another easy way to prepare and cook fennel (anise), to serve as a side dish - Cut fennel In chunks, and drizzle with extra virgin olive oil, salt, pepper, garlic and onion powder and a light sprinkle of grated parmesan cheese, place on a cookie sheet, and bake at 400 degrees for about 30 to 40 minutes. This is a great tasting side dish.

GRAPEFRUIT AND AVOCADO SALAD

Ingredients:

2 pink fresh grapefruit, divided
¼ cup - white vinegar
3 tbsp - honey
¼ tsp - salt
¼ tsp - pepper

1 tsp - vegetable oil
6 cups - mixed salad greens
½ ripe avocado, peeled,
pitted and cut into 1 in. cubes

Instructions:

Peel 1 grapefruit and cut into sections, discard pith. Peel remaining grapefruit, reserve half. Cut remaining grapefruit half into sections, discard pith. Squeeze juice from reserved grapefruit half into a small bowl.

Whisk together grapefruit juice, vinegar, honey, salt and pepper. Add oil, whisking constantly until blended.

Place salad greens on serving platter or in a large bowl. Arrange grapefruit sections over greens. Sprinkle with avocado, and drizzle with dressing.

Nutritional Facts: based on a ½ cup serving

Calories - 120
Sat Fat - 1g
Sodium - 125mg
Carbohydrates - 22g
Protein - 2g

Fat - 4g
Cholesterol - 0g
Potassium - 290mg
Fiber - 3g

COOL SWEET & SPICY CUCUMBER SALAD

Ingredients:

2 English cucumbers, do not peel,
    just slice thin
2 tsp creole seasoning
½ cup - rice wine vinegar

3 tbsp - sugar
½ tsp - crushed red peppers
½ cup - chopped chives

Instructions:

Place cucumber slices in a colander bowl. Sprinkle with creole seasoning; gently toss cucumber slices to coat well. Let stand at room temperature for 15 minutes. Combine the vinegar, sugar and crushed red peppers in another bowl until combined and the sugar has dissolved. Drain the cucumbers and pat dry. Then add the cucumbers to the dressing and blend. Refrigerate for 1 ½ hours and serve chilled. Garnish with chives if desired.

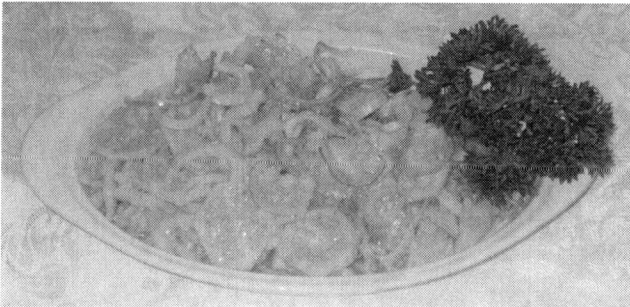

TROPICAL FRUIT SALAD w/
COOL FRUIT VINEGAR DRESSING

Ingredients:

kiwi fruit, peeled and sliced
2 cup fresh pineapple, diced
1 ripe papaya, seeded, peeled and diced
1 ripe mango, peeled, pitted, and diced
¾ cup rice wine vinegar
2 tbsp red onions, chopped
1 cup strawberries, sliced

¼ tsp allspice
1 tbsp honey
½ cup canola oil
salt and pepper - to taste
½ tsp - Mrs. Dash - Table Blend
2 tsp fresh mint leaves, chopped

Instructions:

Place half of kiwi fruit, pineapple, papaya, and mango in a small saucepan. Combine the remaining fruits in a medium boil; cover and refrigerate. Add vinegar to saucepan; cook over medium heat for five (5) minutes or until fruit is softened.

Transfer to refrigerator; chill for 30 minutes. Pour vinegar mixture into a food processor or blender; add onions, honey and allspice. Process until mixture is smooth. With motor running, pour oil through feed tube in a steady stream. Process just until well blended. Season with salt and pepper to taste. Add strawberries, and mint to reserved fruit; toss lightly. Add ½ cup dressing, toss again. Spoon into serving dishes.

Additional suggestions for this fruit dressing: This dressing can also be use as a marinate for chicken or pork, or as a dressing for my green salad with sliced avocado and grapefruit sections.

KUMQUAT SALAD
(AKA Yellow Plums)

Ingredients:

12 Kumquats, thinly sliced
3 tbsp - olive oil
1/8 tsp - cayenne pepper
2 tbsp - raisins (optional)
1 ½ tbsp - balsamic vinegar
¼ tsp - creole seasoning
1 med. - head romaine lettuce, rinsed, dried and cut julienne (thin strips)
1 large - avocado, peeled, quartered, thinly sliced

Instructions:

Heat kumquats in oil and cayenne pepper in a very small skillet over medium heat until you spell a pungent pepper smell.

Add raisins, vinegar and creole seasoning. Cover tightly, and simmer 1-2 minutes. Set aside.

Divide lettuce and avocado on four salad plates

Stir sauce and distribute over salads.

Facts: these beauties from Chinese origin. The skin is pungent and sweet.

Glo's Tip: For a more mellow flavor, drop them into boiling water for 20 seconds. Then drain and chill in ice water. Dry and refrigerate.

Back in the day, down south, when I was in my early teens. During the start of one summer, my sisters and some of my friends took swimming lessons for the first time, and we would take short cuts to the center for lessons, and on the way we would pick fruit from this tree along the way, which we referred to them as yellow plums. Many years later, I was to discover these yellow plums actually had a name (kumquats), and now when I make this fruit Salad, I remember them as yellow plums. Those sure were the good ole' days.

Nutritional Facts: (based on a ½ cup serving)

Calories - 437, carbohydrates - 51g, protein - 28g, cholesterol - 60mg, sodium - 248mg, fiber - 5g, Fat - 14g.

NOTE: **For Potassium - (depending on the avocado used for this particular recipe - if you use a California avocado the potassium for a ½ cup serving is 549mg, and if you use a Florida avocado in this recipe a ½ cup serving is about 742mg.**

WATERCRESS ORZO SALAD

Ingredients:
1 tbsp - olive oil
1 clove garlic - minced
1 cup - Arugula - chopped
1 ½ cup - watercress - chopped
1 ½ cups - orzo pasta - cooked
1 ½ cup - radicchio - julienned
1 tbsp - fresh parsley - chopped
½ tbsp - Creole seasoning
1 tbsp - garlic powder
1 tbsp - onion powder

Instructions:

First bring 3 quarts of water to a boil. Add orzo pasta to Water and stir. Return to a boil and cook, covered 10 to 12 minutes. Remove from heat and drain well in colander. Pour drained pasta into serving bowl. Set aside. Heat oil in a large skillet. Saute garlic, Arugula and watercress over medium heat until wilted slightly. Add pasta and other ingredients to skillet and season to taste with the season all, garlic & onion powder.

Toss well and serve.

Nutritional Facts:

Calories - 167, protein - 3g, carbohydrates - 28g, dietary fiber - 1g, fat - 5g,

GLO'S RENAL FRIENDLY CHEF SALAD

Ingredients:

1 head iceberg lettuce, cut into cubes or Romaine (if you prefer)
Or 2 head of butter lettuce, cut into pieces
4 oz. Low-fat turkey ham, cut into strips or some roasted turkey breast
4 oz. Cooked chicken breast, cut into strips
2 eggs, hard boiled and sliced
½ cup - sun dried tomatoes, chopped
¼ cup radishes, sliced
1 avocado, sliced (optional) - (Dialysis pts: if you need to limit your potassium intake (omit the avocado)
1 tbsp sliced green onion
½ cup - shredded mozzarello cheese

½ cup of French dressing (you can make the French dressing (if you prefer)
From my homemade salad dressing list on page . . . .

Instructions:

In a large salad bowl, combine all eight ingredients mentioned above. Toss, and sprinkle cheese on top. Pour French dressing or my homemade French dressing on top of salad.

When I use to have one of my miserable days of hemo dialysis treatment, this dish is so refreshing and delicious. And now after a night of the cycler alarming and not getting much sleep. (I know you CCPD patients can relate). This dish rejuvenated me.

MEAT TOPPERS

Mango Slaw
Pineapple Relish
Mango Chutney
Balsamic Glazed Onions

HOMEMADE SALSA
AND SEASONINGS RECIPES

Easy Homemade Salsa
Cucumber Avocado Salsa
Papaya Vegetable salsa
Three Fruit Salad
Cabbage and Apple Slaw
Homemade Italian Seasoning
Homemade Taco Seasoning

MEAT TOPPER #1

MANGO SLAW

Ingredients:

1 large ripe fresh mango, peeled and chopped	1 small head cabbage, grated
3 tbsp. Fresh lime juice	½ radicchio, grated
2 tbsp. Canola oil	1 cup - carrots, grated
1 tsp. Salt	2 green onions, thinly sliced
Dash of cayenne pepper	1/3 cup fresh cilantro, chopped

Instructions:

Place mango, lime juice, oil, salt and pepper in a blender; process until smooth and set aside.

Put together cabbage, radicchio, carrot, onions and cilantro in a large bowl; add mango mixture and toss to coat. Chill 30 minutes.

Glo Tip: this slaw is great serve with grilled fish, chicken or pork

Nutritional Facts: (based on ½ cup serving)

Calories - 108, carbohydrates - 16g, protein - 2g, fat - 5g, fiber - 5g, cholesterol - 0mg, Sodium - 420mg

Regarding the potassium intake - for a dialysis pt. ½ cup - carrots - raw - is equivalent to 177mg of potassium, for a ½ cup serving of mango raw - 323mg of potassium and for a ½ cup serving of cabbage - raw - 177mg

MEAT TOPPER #2

PINEAPPLE RELISH

Ingredients:

2 cup - fresh diced pineapple or 2 cup - Crushed pineapple
½ cup - onion chopped
½ cup - red bell pepper, chopped
2 clove - garlic, minced
2 tbsp - fresh mint, chopped
2 tbsp - lemon juice

Glo's Tip: Serve with grilled chicken, steak or seafood.

Instructions:

Place pineapple, onion, red pepper, garlic, mint and lemon juice in a medium bowl. Chill for one (1) hour.

Nutritional Facts: (based on a ½ cup serving)

Calories - 22, carbohydrates - 6g, protein - 0g, fat - 0g, fiber - 1g, cholesterol - 0mg, Sodium - 1mg

For potassium - a ½ cup serving of pineapple is equivalent to 88mg of potassium - diced raw

MEAT TOPPER #3

MANGO CHUTNEY

Ingredients:

2 mangos - chopped in cubes   ½ cup - cilantro - finely chopped
1 papaya - chopped in cubes   1 tbsp - olive oil
1 - finely chopped - red onion   1 tbsp - lemon juice
2 cups - scallions - finely chopped - On an angle - 2 tsp - lemon zest
½ cup - roasted red peppers - finely chopped

Glo's tip: (you can substitute the lemon zest and juice for orange juice and orange zest, if you want a more sweeter tasting chutney)

Instructions:

Mix all these ingredients together, and serve over main meat dish - pork chops, lamb, roasted or baked chicken, etc. etc., - any meat of your choice, it will just spruce up your meat in general.

MEAT TOPPER #4

BALSAMIC GLAZED ONIONS
(GREAT OVER STEAK, CHICKEN OR SEAFOOD)

Ingredients:

4 large red onions, sliced
3 tsp. Extra virgin olive oil
3 tbsp. Balsamic vinegar
½ tsp salt
½ tsp ground black pepper

Instructions:

Put onion slices in bowl and drizzle with oil, vinegar, salt and pepper; toss to coat. Place single layer of aluminum foil-lined baking sheet coated with cooking spray.

Grill onions on medium-heat for 5 to 10 minutes or until onions are tender, stirring occasionally. Remove from grill. Serve with meat or seafood of your choice.

HOMEMADE SALAD DRESSING RECIPES:

Creamy Caesar Style Dressing
Garlic and Herb Dressing
Light French Dressing
Simple Vinegarette Dressing

HOMEMADE SALAD DRESSING RECIPES

HOMEMADE SALAD DRESSING # I - CREAMY CAESAR STYLE DRESSING

Ingredients:

3 clove garlic, minced
2 tsp salt
3 anchovy fillets - finely chopped
1 tsp dry mustard
1 tsp - onion powder
2 tsp worchestire sauce
2 tbsp fresh lemon juice
2 ½ tbsp red wine vinegar
¾ cup olive oil
1 well beaten egg

Instructions:

Put the garlic in a food processor and mince it. Add the salt, anchovy fillets, dry mustard and onion powder and process for 10 seconds. Add the worchestire sauce, lemon juice, and red wine vinegar stir to the processor for 10 minutes. Slowly add the oil, then drizzle in the eggs until the mixture is creamy. Refrigerate. Let dressing stand for half an hour at room temperature before tossing with your choice of vegetables.

HOMEMADE SALAD DRESSING #2 - GARLIC AND HERB DRESSING

Ingredients:

¼ cup - extra virgin olive oil
3 tbsp - red wine vinegar
1 tbsp - white wine
1 tbsp - rice wine vinegar
¼ - ketchup
1 tsp - lemon juice
¼ tsp - worchestire sauce
2 tbsp - garlic minced
1 tsp - Italian herb seasoning
1 tsp - maple syrup

Instructions:

Mix together all the ingredients and refrigerate. Let dressing stand for about 20 minutes at room temperature and toss in the vegetables of your choice.

HOMEMADE SALAD DRESSING #3 - LIGHT FRENCH DRESSING

Ingredients:

½ cup apple cider vinegar or red wine vinegar
½ cup extra virgin olive oil
½ tsp Dijon mustard
3 tbsp shallots - minced
¼ tsp parsley flakes
¼ tsp thyme
¼ tsp basil leaves
¼ tsp celery seeds
A pinch of salt
A pinch of black pepper
2 clove garlic, minced

Instructions:

Mix all ingredients together except the garlic. Pour into a container; add garlic. Let stand at room temperature for at least ½ an hour. Shake well before using.

SIMPLE VINEGARETTE SALAD DRESSING - EXTRA BONUS

When you want a simple salad dressing, (with ingredients that are readily available in you own kitchen)

Ingredients:

4 tbsp - extra virgin olive oil
½ tsp - lime juice
1 tsp - Dijon mustard
1 tsp - ground cumin
1 tsp - creole seasoning
1 tsp - mrs. Dash - table blend
1 tbsp - onion & garlic powder

With a whisk, mix all ingredients together, and toss over romaine lettuce.

EASY HOMEMADE SALSA

Ingredients:

2 tomatoes
1 tsp - garlic, minced
2 tbsp - lemon or lime juice

½ cup - onion, chopped
½ cup - cilantro, chopped

Instructions:

In a food processor or blender. Put all ingredients in the blender and mix, but keep the mixture in a chunky texture. Serve with tortilla chips, homemade tacos, or homemade enchiladas, even fatija.

Nutritional Facts:

Calories - 8
Carbohydrates - 2g
Calcium - 15mg
Fat - 0g
Potassium - 76mg

Protein - 0g
Fiber - 1g
Phosphorus - 9g
Sodium - 5mg
Cholesterol - 0g

CUCUMBER -AVOCADO SALSA

Ingredients:

2 ears of corn, husked
2 tbsp - olive oil
2 cucumbers, seeded
And diced
1 small red onion, diced
2 tomatoes, cored,
Seeded and chopped
1 avocado, peeled, pitted
And chopped

3 tbsp - fresh cilantro,
chopped
jalapeno, seeded and
minced
¼ tsp - finely minced fresh
gingerroot
¼ cup - fresh lime juice
tortilla chips
2 garlic cloves, minced

Instructions:

Preheat grill to medium-high (350 degrees). Brush corn with oil and season with salt and pepper to taste. Grill corn until tender and lightly brown, about 10 minutes, turning occasionally. Remove and let cool. Cut kernels from cob with a smaller bowl placed inside a larger bowl, so that when you remove the kernels, they will collect inside the large bowl. (recipe continues on next page)

Add cucumbers, onion, tomatoes, avocado, garlic, cilantro, jalapeno and ginger. Add lime juice gently, toss to blend the flavors. Chill before serving. Serve with tortilla chips.

Nutritional Facts: based on a ½ cup serving

Calories - 100
Sat Fat - 1g
Potassium - 300mg
Fiber - 3g
Protein - 3g

Fat - 7g
Sodium - 5mg
Carbohydrates - 9g
Sugar - 2g
Omega - 3 - 0g

PAPAYA/VEGETABLE SALSA

Ingredients:

2 ripe papayas

2 jalapeno peppers

1 tbsp - garlic, minced

½ red onion, finely chopped

1 cucumber, peeled, seeded and chopped

½ cup - fresh cilantro, chopped

zest of two limes, grated

½ cup - fresh lime juice

Instructions:

Peel papayas, discard the seeds and cut into ½" cubes. Place the papaya in a bowl. (Wear rubber gloves) - and seed and mince the jalapeno peppers.

Add peppers, garlic, onions, cucumber, cilantro, zest and lime juice. Toss. And Serve

THREE FRUIT SALSA

Ingredients:

1 cup - cantaloupe, chopped

1 cup - mango, chopped

1 cup - strawberries, sliced

½ cup - cucumber, chopped

½ cup - bell pepper, chopped

½ cup - red onion

2 tbsp - jalapeno pepper - minced (optional)

1 tbsp - fresh mint leaves - chopped

1 tbsp - fresh basil leaves - chopped

2 tbsp - fresh lime juice

1 tbsp - honey

1 tsp - creole seasoning

Instructions:

Mix all ingredients in a bowl to combine well. Garnish with whole mint leaves.

Glo's Tip: The salsa is a great compliment to chicken or lamb dishes.

CABBAGE AND APPLE SLAW

Ingredients:

1 lb - shredded cabbage
¼ cup - red onion, chopped
2 - granny smith apples,
Chopped
½ cup - walnuts, chopped

¼ cup - cider vinegar
¼ cup - apple cider or juice
1 ½ tsp - honey
1 ½ tsp - parsley, finely chopped
salt and pepper to taste

Instructions:

In large bowl combine cabbage, onion, apples and walnuts.

For dressing, in small bowl whisk together vinegar cider and honey. Add salt and pepper to taste.

Add dressing to vegetables, and toss. Sprinkle with parsley. Chill until ready to serve.

Nutritional Facts:

Calories - 185
Fat - 9g
Sat Fat - 1g
Cholesterol - 0g
Sodium - 61mg

Potassium - 500mg
Carbohydrates - 24g
Fiber - 5g
Protein - 6g
Omega - 3 - 1g

Note: The phosphorus in cabbage and apples is very low, for walnuts, (black 2 oz - serving - contains 264mg of phosphorus, and 180mg of phosphorus - 2 oz - English) - so be careful with the walnuts, make a sensible choice on how much to use in this recipe, or better yet, omit it all together, to keep Mr. Phosphorus from lurking.

HOMEMADE TACO SEASONING

Ingredients:

3 tbsp - onion powder
2 tbsp - ground cumin
1 ½ tsp - chili powder
½ tsp - cayenne
1 tsp - garlic powder

Instructions:

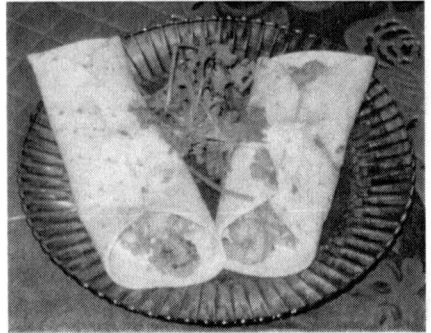

Mix ingredients together and store in an airtight container

Nutritional Facts: based on a 1 tsp - serving

Calories - 6
Fat - 0g
Sodium - 3mg
Calcium - 8mg
Cholesterol - 0mg

Protein - 0g
Carbohydrates - 1g
Potassium - 22mg
Phosphorus - 7mg
Fiber - 0g

HOMEMADE ITALIAN SEASONING

Ingredients:

2 tbsp - garlic powder
1 tbsp - basil, chopped
½ tsp - pepper
2 tsp - onion powder

1 tbsp - parsley, chopped
1 tbsp - dry oregano
½ tsp - dry thyme

Nutritional Fact: based on ½ tsp serving

Calories - 4
Fat - 0g
Sodium - 0mg
Calcium - 6mg

Protein - 0g
Carbohydrates - 1g
Potassium - 16mg
Phosphorus - 4mg

Simple And Easy Soup Recipes

SWEET POTATO SOUP

Ingredients:

3 strips - bacon, cut into ½ in. pieces
½ cup - onion, coarsely chopped
½ cup - carrot, chopped
½ cup - celery, coarsely chopped
1 garlic clove - minced
¼ tsp - salt
1 ½ cup - chicken broth
1 ½ cup - water
2 large - sweet potatoes, peeled and coarsely chopped
1 med. - potato, peeled and coarsely chopped
1/8 tsp - ground nutmeg
½ to 1 ½ cup - milk or (mocha mix to watch the phosphorus intake)

Instructions:

In a large saucepan cook bacon until crisp. Using a slotted spoon, remove bacon, reserving the drippings. Set aside. Drain bacon on paper towels. Cook onion, carrot, celery, garlic and salt in hot drippings for five minutes. Add broth, water, sweet potatoes and potato. If necessary, add additional water to cover vegetables. Bring to boiling; reduce heat. Simmer about 15 minutes or until potatoes are tender. Remove saucepan from heat. Stir in cinnamon and nutmeg.

Pour half of the hot potato mixture into blender container. Cover and blend until smooth, adding enough milk to thin to desired consistency. Pour into serving bowl.

Repeat with remaining mixture. Season to taste with salt and black pepper. Sprinkle each serving with reserved bacon pieces.

Nutritional Facts: based on a ½ cup serving

Calories - 150

Fat - 6g

Sat Fat - 2g

Cholesterol - 10mg

Sodium - 545mg

Potassium - 455mg

Carbohydrates - 21g

Fiber - 3g

Protein - 4g

Omega - 3 - 0g

CREOLE STYLE SEAFOOD SOUP

Ingredients:

1 can - tomato soup
1 cup - half and half or
Mocha mix
8 oz - cooked shrimp, crab meat
And/or lobster meat, cut up

1 tbsp - lemon juice
1 tbsp - fresh chives, chopped
2 tbsp - dry sherry (optional)
2 tsp - fresh chives, chopped

If you want to use homemade tomato soup, I have a homemade recipe to share, check it out.

Instructions:

In a medium saucepan, stir together soup and half and half or mocha mix, if you prefer. Cook over medium heat, stirring often, 5 to 6 minutes or until very hot but not boiling.

Stir in seafood, lemon juice and 1 tbsp - chives. Stir in sherry, if desired. Cook and stir 2 to 4 minutes or until heated through.

Ladle into serving bowls. Sprinkle with remaining 2 tsp chives. Serve immediately.

Nutritional Facts: based on a ½ cup serving

Calories - 180
Sat Fat - 2g
Sodium - 815mg
Carbohydrates - 19g
Protein - 15g

Fat - 5g
Cholesterol - 50mg
Potassium - 290mg
Fiber - 1g

Note: This recipe has a high content of sodium, it is recommended that a dialysis patient has about 2000mg of sodium a day.

MACARONI BRUNSWICK SOUP

Ingredients:

1 tomato, diced
2 cup - cooked okra
2 cup - frozen corn
½ lb. smoked sausage,
Cut into ¼ in. slices
½ tsp - worchestire sauce

1 cup - fried elbow macaroni
2 cup - chicken broth
½ cup - water
½ tsp - ground black pepper
2 cup - chicken or pork, cooked in
Barbeque sauce - about ½ cup

Instructions:

In dutch oven, combine untrained tomatoes, okra, corn, sausage, chicken, macaroni, chicken broth, water, worchestire sauce and pepper.

Bring to a boil. Reduce heat, simmer, uncovered for 20 minutes or until macaroni is tender, stirring frequently.

Nutritional Facts: based on a ½ cup serving

Calories - 330
Carbohydrates - 39g
Fat - 10g
Cholesterol - 46mg
Sodium - 1560mg

Protein - 18g
Fiber - 4g
Sat Fat - 3g
Potassium - 180mg
Omega - 3 - 0g

Glo's tip: Although this is a very tasty soup, beware of the high content of sodium, (it is over the limit for a renal diet, it is recommended that dialysis patients have only 2000mg of sodium a day), so be careful, just know your limits, don't over indulge O.K.

Use low sodium chicken broth in this recipe, to control the sodium in this recipe.

CRANBERRY PESTO

Ingredients:

1 garlic clove
1 cup - dried
Cranberries
1 cup - basil
¼ cup - walnuts,
Toasted

½ cup - parmesan cheese, grated
¼ cup - parsley
¼ cup - olive oil
½ cup - goat cheese
24 unsalted crackers

Instructions:

Pulse garlic in food processor until finely diced, add cranberries, basil, walnuts and paprika, and pulse until blended, but still chunky in texture.

Place mixture in medium bowl; add parmesan, parsley, and oil, and stir well.

Spread 1 tsp - goat cheese over crackers and top with 1 tbsp - of pesto mixture.

Glo's tip: this is great little snack, you can also garnish w/capers, if desired, but remember capers are very salty, so be careful and wise to your sodium intake in your particular renal diet. Also be careful with the walnuts - for a 2 oz serving of black walnuts - there is 264mg of phosphorus, and the English version - 2 oz - 180mg of phosphorus.

HOMEMADE GUACAMOLE

Ingredients:

1 - avocado
Juice of 1 lime
½ tsp - salt
½ tsp - cumin
½ tsp - cayenne

½ - medium onion, diced
2 tomatoes, seeded and diced
1 tbsp - cilantro, chopped
1 garlic clove, minced

Instructions:

Peel one avocado and mash, place in a bowl, Add lime juice, salt, cumin, and cayenne.

Then to bowl, add onion, diced tomatoes, cilantro, and minced garlic, and blend well.

Glo's tip: great in a enchilada, fatija, or taco

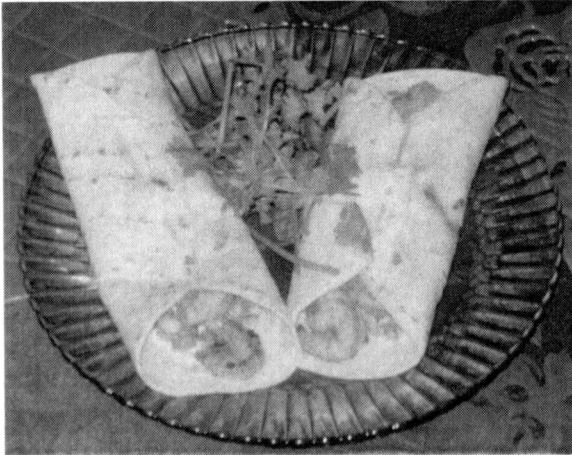

HOMEMADE PESTO

Ingredients:

1 cup - fresh basil leaves
1 head - roasted garlic
2 tbsp - chopped walnuts or pine nuts
4 tbsp - grated parmesan cheese
¼ cup - olive oil

Instructions:

In a food processor, combine basil, garlic, parmesan cheese and nuts. Slowly add olive oil, while machine is still running, process until the ingredients form a paste. Remove pesto and store in a tightly covered container until ready to use.

HERBAL POLENTA

Ingredients:

8 cups - low sodium broth
2 tsp - salt
2 ¼ cups - yellow cornmeal
¾ cup - grated parmesan cheese
4 tbsp - butter or margarine (at room temperature)
½ cup - (fresh rosemary, thyme, parsley, oregano leaves) - finely chopped
½ tsp - black pepper
½ tsp - garlic powder
½ tsp - onion powder

Instructions:

In a medium-size saucepan, bring broth and salt to a boil over high heat. Slowly whisk in cornmeal. When the mixture begins to bubble, reduce the heat to medium-low and cook, stirring until the cornmeal begins to thicken, about 10 to 15 minutes.

Slowly whisk in the remaining ingredients. Continue cooking until the polenta begins to pull away from the sides of the pan, about 3 to 5 minutes.

Serve immediately.

PARMESAN PEARL ONIONS

Ingredients:

1 pkg - fresh pearl onions
½ cup - parmesan cheese, grated
½ cup - half and half
1/8 tsp - pepper
1 tsp - garlic powder

1 tbsp - flour
½ tsp - salt
½ tsp - worchestire sauce
1/8 tsp - paprika

Instructions:

Cook onions in boiling water for a couple of minutes; remove onions from water and plunge into ice water; peel.

Arrange onions in lightly greased 1-quart baking dish and sprinkle with parmesan cheese.

Preheat oven to 300 degrees. Combine half and half, flour, salt, worchestire sauce, garlic powder and pepper; stir well and bake 15 minutes or until tender. Serve with slotted spoon.

Nutritional Facts: based on a 2 oz serving

Calories - 118
Sat Fat - 4g
Sodium - 580mg
Carbohydrates - 7g
Protein - 6g

Fat - 7g
Cholesterol - 25mg
Potassium - 20mg
Fiber - 0g
Omega - 3 - 0g

Note: parmesan cheese as 229mg of phosphorus in a 1 oz - serving, it falls in the highest category of the food finder chart, so be careful with your phosphorus intake in this recipe.

BRAISED FENNEL WITH CARAMELIZED ONIONS

Ingredients:

1 large - red onion, thinly sliced
1 tbsp - balsamic vinegar
¾ cup - low sodium chicken broth

1 tbsp - olive oil
2 med - fennel bulbs
2 tbsp - walnuts or pine nuts (optional)

Instructions:

In skillet cook onion in olive oil over low heat, stirring frequently 5 minutes. Cover and cook 10 minutes more, stirring occasionally or until onions are very tender and edges are golden. Add balsamic vinegar and cook and stir until onions are coated.

Meanwhile, trim fennel; chip enough of green tops to make 2 tsp, set aside. Cut each fennel bulb lengthwise into six wedges. In medium size saucepan cook fennel wedges, covered, in chicken broth for 10 to 12 minutes or until tender. Drain.

Arrange fennel wedges on serving plate. Top with onions and sprinkle with nuts and reserved fennel tops.
Note: At my neighborhood farmers market, fennel is called anise.

Nutritional Facts: based on a ½ cup serving

Calories - 110
Sat Fat - 1g
Sodium - 60mg
Carbohydrates - 12g
Protein - 3g
Fat - 7g
Cholesterol - 0mg
Potassium - 520mg
Fiber - 4g

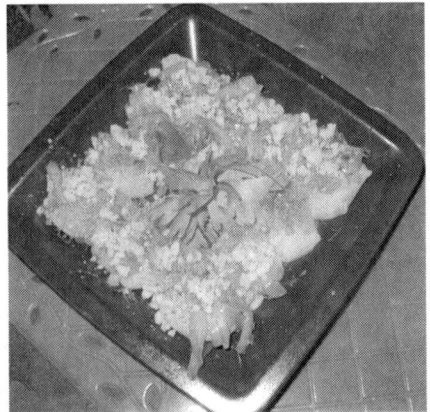

SIMPLE AND EASY TOMATO SOUP

Ingredients:

2 tbsp - unsalted margarine   1 cup - chicken broth
1/3 cup - onion, chopped   1 cup - heavy cream
1 (28 oz) - can diced tomatoes

Instructions:

Melt margarine in a 3-quart heavy bottomed saucepan. Add onions and saute" for 2 minutes. Add tomatoes, chicken broth and cream to onions. Bring to a boil, reduce heat, and simmer 5 minutes.

Pour into a blender or food processor. Blend until smooth. Pour into soup bowls.

Glo's tip: garnish with sour cream, it is great as a topping

DESSERTS

7-UP CAKE

Ingredients:

1 ½ cup - tub margarine	3 cup - sugar
5 eggs	3 cup - flour
2 tsp - lemon or vanilla extract	¾ cup - 7-up

Instructions:

Preheat oven to 325 degrees. Cream margarine and sugar together and beat until light and fluffy. Add eggs, one at a time and beat well, and then add flour. Add in lemon and 7-up.

Pour batter into well-greased and floured bundt pan.

Bake for 1 ¼ hour, when cool, top with sifted powdered sugar.

Nutritional Facts: based on a 1/12 piece

Calories - 416	Sodium - 201mg
Protein - 5g	Potassium - 54mg
Fat - 19g	Calcium - 18mg
Carbohydrates - 57g	Phosphorus - 63mg
Fiber - 1g	Cholesterol - 124mg

KEYLIME PIE

Ingredients:

Six (6) - Egg yolks
1 can - sweetened condensed milk
2 tbsp - lime zest
¾ cup - lime juice
½ tsp - lemon extract
Whip cream for topping
Coconut sprinkles - (optional) - for topping
One ready made graham cracker crust

Instructions:

First mix the six yolks, then add the milk, lime zest, lime juice and lemon extract. Pour egg mixture in the graham cracker crust.

Set in freezer for two hours.

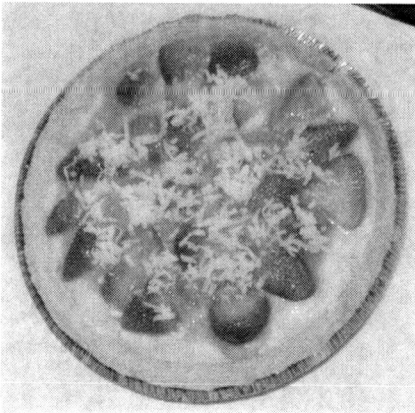

DOWNHOME CORNBREAD

Ingredients:

1 cup - cornmeal
1 cup - all-purpose flour

1 tsp - baking powder
½ tsp - baking soda
1 cup of buttermilk

2 eggs, slightly beaten
¼ of melted butter, or tub - margarine
(dialysis pts.)
2 tbsp - sugar
2 tbsp - salt

Instructions:

Pre-heat oven for 425 F.

In a large bowl, mix the dry ingredients together (cornmeal, flour, baking powder, soda, sugar, and salt).
Then add the butter.

Coat the bottom of a cast iron skillet with the olive oil or butter spray and pour the cornmeal mixture in the skillet and place in the oven and bake for 20-25 minutes or until golden brown.

SOUTHERN STYLE BLACKBERRY COBBLER

Ingredients:

3 cups - fresh or frozen
Blackberries
3 tbsp - cornstarch
1 tbsp - tub margarine

1 cup - sugar
¼ tsp - ground cinnamon
1 cup - cold water

Instructions:

In a large saucepan, combine the blackberries, sugar, and cinnamon. Cook and stir until mixture comes to a boil. Combine the cornstarch and water until smooth; stir into fruit mixture. Bring to a boil, cook and stir for 2 minutes or until thickened. Pour into a greased 8-in. square baking dish, and dot with butter or margarine.

BISCUIT TOPPING:

1 ½ cups - all purpose flour
1 ½ tsp - baking powder
½ cup - cold butter or margarine
½ cup - 2% milk or mocha mix (to watch the phosphorous intake)
Whipped topping or vanilla ice cream (optional)

1 tbsp - sugar
½ tsp - salt

Instructions:

In a small bowl, combine the flour, sugar, baking powder and salt. Cut in margarine until mixture resembles coarse crumbs. Stir in milk or mocha mix, just until moistened. Drop by tablespoonfuls onto hot berry-mixture.

Bake, uncovered, at 350F for 30-35 minutes or until filling is bubbly and topping is golden brown. Serve warm with whipped topping or ice cream.

Nutritional Facts: based on a 1/12 piece

Cooked from raw - ½ cup - blackberries

Protein - 1g   Sodium - 2mg   Potassium - 141mg
Phosphorus - 15mg   Calories - 37

Cooked from frozen - ½ cup - blackberries
Protein - 0.5g   Sodium - 1mg   Potassium - 105mg
Phosphorus - 23mg   Calories - 69

A childhood memory to share:

I remember when my sisters and some friends and I would go to the woods, to pick blackberries, and when we would come to a leaf that had a spit like substance on it, we would run like the dickens, because we were told that when we would see this spit on a leave, that meant that a snake had visited there, but I don't know from this day, how true that was, but we kids would look out for those kinds of leaves.

I think about this time, when I would purchase blackberries at my neighborhood farmers market, and say to myself, I never thought I would be buying blackberries today, those sure were the good old days, when everything was carefree.

PAPAYA POUND CAKE TOPPING

Ingredients:

1 large papaya, halved,
Seeded, peeled and cut
Into cubes
1 tsp - finely grated
¼ cup - lime juice
And zest of 1 lime

Instructions:

Toss papaya with lime peel, lime juice and honey in a large bowl. Let stand 15 minutes. Make this homemade pound 7-UP cake recipe and top the papaya mixture on top, the recipe for the 7UP Pound Cake is on page - 249 . . . .

APPLE CRANBERRY CRUNCH

Ingredients:

6 med - apple, cored, peeled and sliced
2 cups - fresh or frozen cranberries
¾ cup - sugar
½ tsp - cinnamon

Instructions:

In a large bowl, combine apples, cranberries, sugar, and cinnamon. Put apple-cranberry mixture into 13X9 in. Baking dish. Sprinkle Topping evenly over Filling. Bake at 375 degrees for 1 hour.

Topping:

¼ cup - flour
¼ cup - dry oat meal
¼ cup - brown sugar
¼ tsp - ginger
¼ tsp - nutmeg
3 tbsp - canola oil
1 tbsp - honey

Instructions:

mix flour, oats, brown sugar, ginger and nutmeg. Add oil, and honey, mix well to make coarse crumbs

Nutritional Facts: based on 1/12 serving

Calories - 169
Fat - 4g
Fiber - 2g
Potassium - 120mg
Phosphorus - 27mg

Protein - 1g
Carbohydrates - 34g
Sodium - 2mg
Calcium - 11mg
Cholesterol - 0g

Making Gravy - A simple gravy can be made from 2 tbsp - of butter or tub margarine for dialysis pts. - with 2 tbsp of flour, make into a paste and add chicken broth, or stock and stir until you get the right consistency, and then pour a dot of kitchen bouquet for flavor and color desired, the more kitchen bouquet you add in, the more richer and darker the roux or gravy becomes.

Pan dripping Gravy - After cooking your meat, pour a tbsp of red wine and scrap the bottom of the pan, where those burnt like bits and pieces lie, (they have great flavor), in the pan juices, then whisk 2 tbsp of flour and butter or margarine together. (if needed slowly add a little chicken stock or broth, until mixture appear smooth, then add a dot of kitchen bouquet for flavor and color.

How to Roast Garlic - Cut the head of the garlic off - about ¼ in. from root end. Place exposed end up, cover with aluminum foil and drizzle a little olive oil on top, place on cookie sheet and bake on 375 f for about 15 to 20 minutes, depending on your oven.

Simple Instructions for Oven Fried Bacon:

Preheat oven for 400 F. Layer Bacon on a Cookie Sheet and Bake until crispy about 15 to 20 minutes.

How to make an easy viniagerette dressing for a simple green salad?

Ingredients: In a bowl, the juice of one lemon, 1 tbsp - red wine vinegar, 1 tsp - Dijon mustard, a dash of worchestire sauce, ½ cup - extra virgin olive oil, 1 tsp - garlic powder, 1 tsp - onion powder and 2 anchovies - minced (optional). Whisk all ingredients together, except the olive oil, whisk slowly at the end. Pour over a bed of romaine, Arugula, or watercress (whatever is your preference).

Glo's tip on how to help the produce last longer.

Having only three people living in the household, produce can go bad real fast, so I decided to conduct a little experiment. I purchased those Debbie's green bags, and plus aluminum foil. I discovered that wrapping my fruits and vegetables in aluminum foil, they stay fresh much longer, and I don't have to continue throwing away fruit and vegetables that have gone bad, and with the economy being weak, I had to find a compromise to all this. Now, I have a large investment in aluminum foil and Debbie green bags. I also keep my green onion fresh for a long period of time. I just cut the whites from the green, and wrap them separate in aluminum foil and place it in the green bags. I have done pretty good so far, this summer, just wanted to share that little tip with you readers.

How to make a simple and easy potato salad?

Ingredients:

1 bag of frozen O-gratin potatoes
2 eggs - hard boiled and crumbled

1 tsp - garlic powder
1 tsp - onion powder
1 tsp - creole seasoning
1 tsp - Mrs. Dash
(table blend) seasoning
½ cup - mayonnaise

1 tbsp - mustard
1 tbsp - rice wine vinegar or
white wine vinegar
2 tbsp - sweet pickled relish
½ cup - celery - chopped
½ tsp - garlic salt
½ cup - shallots - chopped
½ cup - green onions
(with scallions) - chopped

Instructions:

1. Put the frozen potatoes in a bowl w/a damp paper towel placed over it. Then place in micro wave oven for about 2 minutes.
2. Meanwhile hard boil two eggs. Crumble the eggs in a bowl, then add the garlic powder, onion powder, creole seasoning, garlic salt and Mrs. Dash.
3. To the potatoes, fold the egg seasoning mixture, then the mayonnaise, mustard, vinegar, relish, celery, shallots, and green onions. Mix well. Serve at room temperature.

Homemade High Protein Drinks

Note: From time to time a dialysis patient may have low protein, (especially peritoneal dialysis patients, who lose protein more easily) may need to add more protein to their diet, but if you can't achieve this through your renal diet, then a protein supplement maybe prescribed for you, or you can try some of the following protein drink recipes (that are very easy to make and very beneficial in obtaining more protein in your diet).

High Protein Drink Recipes

SORBET SMOOTHIE

FRUIT SMOOTHIE
(IDEAL FOR A DIABETIC/RENAL DIET)

HIGH PROTEIN SMOOTHIE

PEACH HIGH PROTEIN FRUIT SMOOTHIE

SORBET SMOOTHIE

Ingredients:

2 eggs
½ cup - sorbet (any flavor of your choice)

Instructions:

Put eggs and sorbet in a blender, and blend for 30 seconds. Pour in a cup and drink immediately. You can freeze the remaining smoothie mix. Remove from freezer ½ hour before drinking to de-thaw.

To make this high protein drink friendly for diabetics, the recipe as follows:

2 cups - egg substitute
½ cup - sorbet (any flavor of your choice)

Follow same instructions as the regular sorbet smoothie recipe above

Facts: Egg substitutes (like Egg beaters) are safe to use uncooked and the perfect base ingredient to make a high protein smoothie.

Fact: Each ½ cup - egg beater has 12 grams of protein

Nutritional Info:

130 calories, 15 grams - carbohydrates, 12 grams - protein per one (1) cup serving, ideal for diabetics.

Glo's Tip: Try blending egg substitute with; mocha mix, low potassium fruit such as:

Blueberries - ½ cup serving - raw - 65 mg
Cranberries - ½ cup serving - raw - 39 mg
Pineapple - ½ cup serving - raw - 88 mg
Raspberries - ½ cup serving - raw - 94 mg

Watermelon - ½ cup serving - 93 mg
Strawberries - ½ cup serving - 124 mg - (from the higher mg list)
Peaches - 1 medium - diced - 171 mg - (from the higher mg list)
Pears - 1 medium - diced - 148 mg - (from the higher mg list)

Glo's tip: You can also blend egg substitute with diet sherbet, sorbet, and nutrasweet, for a great tasting high protein drink.

FRUIT SMOOTHIE RECIPE
(This recipe is great for diabetics)

Ingredients:

1 cup - egg substitute (such as egg beater or better n eggs)
1 cup - fat free mocha mix
½ cup - strawberries
1-2 packages of nutrasweet

Instructions:

Blend all ingredients in blender for 30 seconds and serve chilled.

Glo's Tip: You can use other fresh fruits like pineapple, blueberries, and raspberries.

HIGH PROTEIN SMOOTHIE

Ingredients:

1 small carton (1 ounce) - frozen strawberries, lightly sweetened
1/3 can (6 oz. Can) - frozen pineapple juice concentrate
½ cup - pasteurized egg whites (or 2 egg whites)
1 scoop - (approx. 1/3 cup) whey protein powder
2 tbsp - nondairy whipped topping

Instructions:

First, blend egg whites in a blender for 2 minutes. Second, add strawberries, pineapple concentrate and protein powder, blend at medium speed until smooth. Third, pour 1/3 cup of the smoothie into a glass and top with whipped topping if desired. Fourth, store the remainder in the refrigerator (1 day) or freezer to enjoy later.

Nutritional fact: there is about 152 calories per serving, about 9 grams of protein, 27 grams of carbohydrates, 1 gram of fat, 10 mg of cholesterol, 74 mg of sodium, 302 mg of potassium, 70 mg of phosphorus, 95 mg of calcium and 1.5 grams of fiber.

Glo's tip: the protein powder can be increased to 2 scoops for a higher protein smoothie. Pasteurized egg whites are recommended to avoid the risk of salmonella. Look for refrigerated egg whites in a carton in the dairy section, or dried eggs whites in the baking section at your local grocery store.

PEACH HIGH-PROTEIN FRUIT SMOOTHIE

Ingredients:

¼ cup water (or ½ cup - ice)
2 tbsp - powdered egg whites
¾ cup - peaches (fresh or frozen)
1 tbsp - sugar (or artificial sweetener to taste)

Instructions:

Place peaches in blender and blend until smooth.
Add all remaining ingredients and continue blending until smooth.

Nutritional facts:

There is about 132 calories in this drink, 10 grams of protein, 24 grams of carbohydrates, 0% of fat, no cholesterol, 154 mg of sodium, 353 mg of potassium, 36 mg of phosphorus, 9 mg of calcium, and 1.9 grams of fiber.

Glo's Tip: you can substitute the peaches for ¾ cup of strawberries

Nutritional Facts for Strawberries is slightly different than peaches, there is about 155 mg of sodium, 277 mg of potassium, 25 mg of phosphorus, 18 mg of calcium and 2.3 grams of fiber. No fat, or cholesterol, same as with peaches, as well as the protein and carbohydrates are same as the peaches.

Glo's tip: Also if you like jello, try making your next batch and add a protein powder to it.

HIGH PROTEIN GELATIN CUPS

Ingredients:

1 small box of gelatin   1 cup - whey protein powder
¾ cup boiling water   ¾ cup - cold water

Instructions:

Dissolve gelatin in the boiling water and then dissolve the protein powder in the cold water. After the protein powder is completely dissolved, combine the gelatin mixture with the protein powder mixture.

Pour the mixture in 2-ounce cups and refrigerate until jelled.

Nutritional Facts:

Calories - 58   Fat - 0 grams   Potassium - 34 mg
Protein - 6 grams   Cholesterol - 5 mg   Phosphorus - 34 mg
Carbohydrate - 8 grams   Sodium - 33 mg   Calcium - 38 mg
Fiber - 0 grams

BREADCRUMBS:

Ideas for Breadcrumbs - With a food processor you can make all kinds of breadcrumbs, here are some breadcrumb ideas that I create when I don't have any on hand.

You can make breadcrumb from just about any chips, or crackers, wheat thin, etc. etc.,

1 can - fried onions
½ cup - parsley
1 tbsp - ground ginger
1 tbsp - garlic and onion seasoning

Instruction: In a food processor, mix all ingredients together to breadcrumb consistency.

2 cups - Sun chips
¼ cup - grated parmesan cheese
1/3 cup - parsley

I also make breadcrumbs, from left over French bread., just put it in the food processor and grind it to fine breadcrumb consistency.

Note: Same Instructions as the Fried Onion Breadcrumbs

Recipe for turning crackers into breadcrumb

2/½ cups - unsalted crackers
¼ cup - grated parmesan cheese
2 garlic cloves
½ seeded and ribs removed jalapeno pepper

Glo's tip: just be creative with making your breadcrumbs, add herbs and spices to enhance the flavor of the breadcrumbs, of course, with meat, you may not need to season the meat, because the breadcrumbs will make the meat very tasty.

BREADS AND CEREALS

Foods in this list are good sources of calories and are fairly low in potassium. However, breads and starches contain a significant amount of protein and need to be considered in your total daily protein intake. Products identified in this list may vary extensively according to brand.

Glo's tip: Remember to read labels for protein, sodium and potassium content when available, and be very wise to a content of phosphorus in these products.

Here is a breakdown of nutritional facts about varies breads

Bagel - based on ½ serving
Protein - 3.5gm   phosphorus - 30mg
Sodium - 150mg   Calories - 90
Potassium - 32mg

French Bread - based on a 1 slice serving
Protein - 3gm   Phosphorus - 30mg
Sodium - 203mg   Calories - 102
Potassium - 32mg

English Muffin - ½ serving
Protein - 2.5gm   Phosphorus - 34mg
Sodium - 189mg   Calories - 70
Potassium - 165mg

Pita - ½ serving
Protein - 2gm   Phosphorus - 19mg
Sodium - 107mg   Calories - 53
Potassium - 22mg

Raisin - 1 slice
Protein - 2gm   Phosphorus - 25
Sodium - 103mg   Calories - 14
Potassium - 66mg
Rye - 1 slice - light
Protein - 2.5gm   Phosphorus - 42mg

Sodium - 103mg   Calories - 69
Potassium - 41mg

Sour dough bread - 1 slice
Protein - 3gm   Phosphorus - 30mg
Sodium - 203mg   Calories - 102
Potassium - 32mg

Tortilla, corn - based on 1 serving
Protein - 1gm   Phosphorus - 29mg
Sodium - 28mg   Calories - 36
Potassium - 28mg

Tortilla, flour - 1 serving
Protein - 3gm   Phosphorus - 23mg
Sodium - 127mg   Calories - 123
Potassium - 26mg

White Bread - 1 slice
Protein - 2.5gm   Phosphorus - 27mg
Sodium - 144mg   Calories - 77
Potassium - 30mg

Whole wheat bread - 1 slice
Protein - 3gm   Phosphorus - 65mg
Sodium - 149mg   Calories - 69
Potassium - 77mg

Hamburger Buns - 1 count
Protein - 3gm   Sodium - 202mg
Potassium - 35mg   Phosphorus - 34mg
Calories - 119

Dinner Rolls - 1 count
Protein - 25mg   Sodium - 142mg
Potassium - 27mg   Phosphorus - 24mg
Calories - 83

BREAKFAST FOODS:

I've never been a big breakfast person, and I know it is said to be the most important meal of the day. I usually eat a couple of boiled eggs, (without the yolk, to cut down on my cholesterol intake) and some kind of fruit cut up and marinated with balsamic vinegar, and sometime I would bake some blueberry muffins and have one with some cut up fruit, and on occasion I would have grits, scrambled eggs and yes, bacon, but I don't over indulge, it is OK to have a couple of strips of bacon with your breakfast. Eating breakfast, as I am aware, will help to jump-start the metabolism and will also help to burn calories throughout the day.

I also from time to time, will eat a bowl of cereal, with some cut up fruits, such as blackberries, raspberries, blue berries, strawberries or cantaloupe or watermelon, which you need to be careful of the potassium intake, just beware of your particular limits of these fruits. I eat the cereal by snacking on them, straight out of the box, I tried mocha mix with them, but I don't particularly like the mocha mix with my cereal, and of course, milk is totally out, because of the phosphorus intake, so yes, I snack on them, just dry cereal, and believe it or not, I don't even miss the milk. I have discovered that as a snack they are great. See, how much the renal diet has changed my way of eating.

Here is a small list of nutritional values of some of my favorite breakfast foods:

Blueberry Muffin - based on a 1 serving
Protein - 2.5gm   Sodium - 200mg
Potassium - 48mg   Phosphorus - 80mg
Calories - 126

Danish - 1 serving
Protein - 2.5gm   Sodium - 132mg
Potassium - 55mg   Phosphorus - 38mg
Calories - 147mg

Doughnut - cake - 1
Protein - 1gm   Sodium - 139mg

Potassium - 27mg

Phosphorus - 55mg

Calories - 105

Doughnut - yeast - 1

Protein - 1gm

Sodium - 99mg

Potassium - 34mg

Phosphorus - 32mg

Calories - 176

Sweet Roll - without nuts - 1

Protein - 5gm

Sodium - 238mg

Potassium - 73mg

Phosphorus - 71mg

Calories - 274

CEREAL - COOKED - NO SALT ADDED

Cream of what - based on ½ cup serving

Protein - 2gm

Sodium - 1mg

Potassium - 4mg

Phosphorus - 40mg

Calories - 67

Farina - ½ cup serving

Protein - 2gm

Sodium - 1mg

Potassium - 6mg

Phosphorus - 17mg

Calories - 70

Grits - ½ cup serving

Protein - 2gm

Sodium - 1mg

Potassium - 13mg

Phosphorus - 12mg

Calories - 61

Hot cereals:

Oatmeal - based on a ½ cup serving

Protein - 3gm

Sodium - 1mg

Potassium - 65mg

Phosphorus - 79mg

Calories - 74

Oat Bran - ½ cup

Protein - 3gm

Sodium - 1mg

Potassium - 90mg   Phosphorus - 100mg
Calories - 45

Cereal - cold - ready to eat
Cheerios - based on a 1 ¼ cup serving
Protein - 4gm   Sodium - 320mg
Potassium - 94mg   Phosphorus - 120mg
Calories - 112

Corn flakes - 1 cup
Protein - 2gm   Sodium - 294mg
Potassium - 34mg   Phosphorus - 11mg
Calories - 108

Fruit Loops - 1 cup
Protein - 2gm   Sodium - 127mg
Potassium - 31mg   Phosphorus - 28mg
Calories - 110

Grape nut - 1/3 cup
Protein - 5gm   Sodium - 231mg
Potassium - 99mg   Phosphorus - 79mg
Calories - 138

Honey Smacks - 1 cup
Protein - 2gm   Sodium - 94mg
Potassium - 53mg   Phosphorus - 47mg
Calories - 147

Puffed Rice - based on a 2 cup serving
Protein - 2gm   Sodium - 1mg
Potassium - 30mg   Phosphorus - 51mg
Calories - 110

Puff Wheat - 1 cup
Protein - 2gm   Sodium - 1mg
Potassium - 47mg   Phosphorus - 48mg
Calories - 54

Raisin bran - 1 cup
Protein - 5gm   Sodium - 302mg
Potassium - 312mg   Phosphorus - 201mg
                                Calories - 169

Rice krispies - 1 cup
Protein - 2gm   Sodium - 340mg
Potassium - 29mg   Phosphorus - 28mg
Calories - 117

Shredded wheat - based on a 1 biscuit serving
Protein - 2.5gm   Sodium - 1mg
Potassium - 87mg   Phosphorus - 97mg
Calories - 89

COOKIES: (SNACK TREAT) - And remember to take some binders with these snacks as well.

Here is a breakdown of nutritional values of my favorite snacks

Ginger Snaps - based on 2 cookie serving
Protein - 1gm   Sodium - 80mg
Potassium - 65mg   Phosphorus - 7mg
Calories - 59

Short Bread Cookies - 3 cookie serving
Protein - 1.5gm   Sodium - 14mg
Potassium - 15mg   Phosphorus - 35mg
Calories - 112

Homemade Sugar Cookies - 1.3" diam. Serving
Protein - 0.5gm   Sodium - 34mg
Potassium - 8mg   Phosphorus - 11mg
Calories - 47

Sugar Wafers - 5 serving
Protein - 2gm   Sodium - 90mg
Potassium - 29mg   Phosphorus - 38mg

Calories - 230

Vanilla Wafers - 5 serving
Protein - 1gm   Sodium - 50mg
Potassium - 14mg   Phosphorus - 13mg
Calories - 92

CRACKERS:

Graham - based on a 3 square serving
Protein - 1.5gm   Sodium - 141mg
Potassium - 81mg   Phosphorus - 31mg
Calories - 81

Rye krisp - 4 serving
Protein - 3gm   Sodium - 412mg
Potassium - 64mg   Phosphorus - 78mg
Calories - 96

FLOUR:

All purpose flour - based on a 2 tbsp serving
Protein - 3gm   Sodium - 0mg
Potassium - 14mg   Phosphorus - 12mg
Calories - 96

PASTA: based on a ½ cup serving

Egg noodles
Protein - 3gm   Sodium - 2mg
Potassium - 35mg   Phosphorus - 47mg
Calories - 100

Spaghetti
Protein - 2.5gm   Sodium - 1mg
Potassium - 43mg   Phosphorus - 35mg

Calories - 78

Macaroni
Protein - 2.5gm   Sodium - 1mg
Potassium - 43mg   Phosphorus - 35mg
Calories - 78

SNACKS: Portions as stated

Graham cracker - 3 squares
Protein - 1.5gm   Sodium - 141mg
Potassium - 81mg   Phosphorus - 31mg
Calories - 81

Rye-krisp - 4 count
Protein - 3gm   Sodium - 412mg
Potassium - 64mg   Phosphorus - 78mg
Calories - 96

Popcorn - 2 cup serving - plain, popped
Protein - 1.5gm   Sodium - 0mg
Potassium - 31mg   Phosphorus - 34mg
Calories - 46

Pretzels - 1 oz. serving
Protein - 2gm   Sodium - 378mg
Potassium - 29mg   Phosphorus - 29mg
Calories - 88

Corn chips - 1 oz serving - unsalted (about 11 chips)
Protein - 2gm   Sodium - 10mg
Potassium - 65mg   Phosphorus - 5mg
Calories - 139

White Rice - based on ½ cup serving
Protein - 2gm   Sodium - 0mg
Potassium - 29mg   Phosphorus - 29mg
Calories - 112

All purpose flour - based on 2 tbsp.

Protein - 3gm   Sodium - 0mg

Potassium - 14mg   Phosphorus - 12mg

Calories - 96

What Helps Me Live A Joyful Life
In Spite of Kidney Disease

In the beginning when I was first diagnose with end stage renal disease, I was working a nine to five job and raising my toddler daughter as a single parent, I must admit at first I was in denial, although in the early 70's during my dad's ordeal with the polycystic kidney disease and hemo dialysis of course, he would talk to me during his treatment, and talk about this polycystic kidney disease and how it has plagued our family in a big way. And when this finally hit me in my early thirties, I was told by my neprologist that within five years of giving birth to my premature daughter from complications of preclampsia, and of course the inheritance of the polycystic kidney disease, that it would be inevitable that I would develop end stage renal disease within that timeframe, and dialysis or transplantation was the end result. Well it took me many months to find joy in all this, and what I do credit my joyous outlook on, is my daughter, (the most important part of my existence), she is what kept me grounded and leveled headed coping with this life, which helped me to accept it and embrace it. Another joyous part of this life, has given me some sense of direction and appreciation for my life. I finally this year made an accomplishment a reality, I self-published a book about my 20 years of living my life coping with the polycystic kidney disease and dialysis treatment. I felt so much confidence and joy writing my memoirs of trials and tribulations embracing this new life, it was very therapeutic for me. It gave me such pleasure to share what I know and have endured living in the renal world. Living on Dialysis, I've matured so much more, I don't take anything for granted anymore. I have even taken up crafting, in which I don't think I would have ever adopted as a hobby if I wasn't a dialysis patient. I feel my lifestyle has gotten very unique since becoming a dialysis patient. I truly find pleasure in simple things, like being fortunate enough to live in the backyard of the most beautiful country side. My husband takes me on long country drives through the Napa and Sonoma wine country very often, this truly gives me peace of mind, I even forget about my aches and pains at one point. Although mind over matter doesn't last very long with me, because I don't do very well with pain. The routine is after the country drive, we would drop by our favorite neighborhood Farmer's Market (Larry's Produce), and of course I am all smiles looking at the wonderful abundance of fruits and vegetables that the market provides and my smile gets even more pronounced when I see those very affordable prices. I also get a chance to see some of my fellow hemo dialysis patients outside the unit at the market, and sometime we exchange cooking tips. I also like to frequent the 99 cent store for fresh produce, especially asparagus and some other products, (such as: low sodium chicken broth, and on occasion I purchase smoke salmon) Isn't that something!. Well anyway, this really gives me a sense of inner peace, especially since we are living in a weak economy these days, I can still make gourmet meals for my family and I, and I don't have to worry about not being able to continue eating nutritious and healthy meals that will accommodate my renal diet needs. But you know what really puts a big smile on my face, its when my PD nurse can draw my blood on the first try, I swear I could truly kiss her on the jaw, because being a dialysis patient for as long as I have been one, my veins are not as friendly anymore. And it goes the same for getting an IV, I sit still and pray that they can get my IV on the first try, but of course that rarely ever happens, it usually takes two to three tries. And of course going to church, it keeps me in the reality of appreciating the life that I have, regardless of my kidney disease. I think about something my mom would always say, "Even though you may have pain you think you can't bare, just remember you will never suffer as much as Jesus did".

When a patient with chronic kidney disease, develops Stage - 5 (End Stage Renal Disease), a form of dialysis or the blessing of a transplant, becomes absolutely necessary for continued survival. And just remember, Dialysis or Transplantation is not a cure, they are still a form of treatment for end stage renal disease. First let's get acquainted with the abbreviations or short term of these particular form of dialysis treatment. Hemodialysis is often referred to in the Dialysis World as Hemo or HD. There is also another form of hemo done at home - often referred to as HHD (Home Hemodialysis) (NX Stage), and finally there is Peritoneal Dialysis, often referred to as PD, and also home dialysis.

HEMODIALYSIS VS. PERITONEAL DIALYSIS

How the treatment methods are done:

Hemodialysis is done by using a machine (an artificial kidney/filter) to remove the Toxins and excess fluids.

Peritoneal Dialysis uses the peritoneum (an area behind The abodmen), which has a Natural filter, a semi-permeable Membrane to remove the toxins And excess fluids.

Note: Both treatments require the blood to be filtered and excess fluids to be removed.

The access of both form of dialysis treatment:

In order to achieve this with Hemodialysis, you need to have an access, such as a fistula or graft, which is a minor surgery to be placed under the skin, although under the skin, it is a very noticeable appearance.

In order to achieve this with Peritoneal Dialysis, a minor surgery, to have a catherer in place in the belly, which 5 inches of the catherer is however very visible outside the body.

Where the treatment is done for each form of dialysis:

Hemodialysis, requires the patient to stick to a Schedule and go to a

Peritoneal Dialysis, can be done at home or elsewhere, at the time facility to have their Treatment.   that's best for the patient.

Advantages of Both Treatments:

Traveling - Hemodialysis requires advance planning for a visiting dialysis facility

Peritoneal Dialysis - gives the patient the freedom of travel with no pre-arranging of treatment in a facility where the patient are vacationing.

Disadvantages of each treatment:

Hemodialysis, - requires the patient to be stuck with two (2) needles at each treatment.

Peritoneal Dialysis - puts the patient at a higher risk for infection, the possible development of a umbilical hernia from the dwelling of the dialysate overtime.

Advantages of both treatments:

Hemodialysis, - is done by the staff with little help from the patient, but the patient can chose to be more involved in the care of their treatment, if they prefer.

Peritoneal Dialysis, - is done by the patient at home requiring the changing of dialysate bags four (4) times per day, (which can get tiring and tedious at times). Peritoneal Dialysis requires training for a couple of weeks to learn how to do the peritoneal dialysis properly. However, a longer overnight treatment is also an option, after the patient has become comfortable with doing the manual PD at home.

The Schedule required to following both treatments:

Hemodialysis, - is usually done three times a week - either Monday, Wednesday, Friday, or Tuesday, Thursday, Saturday - with two days in between with a break from treatment.

Peritoneal Dialysis, - is required every day

Dietary Requirements for each treatment:

Hemodialysis, - requires a great deal of dietary restrictions

Peritoneal Dialysis, - allows for more freedom regarding food and drink intake, but of course there are cases where some patients may have issues with protein and potassium, such as myself, who struggles with this from time to time, because I lose an excessive amount of protein and potassium at each exchange, but don't fret! There are solutions, if this ever arises, by eating more protein and potassium, but if that can't be achieved, a potassium supplement could be prescribed and for the protein, there are protein products on the market, such as protein drinks, protein bars and protein whey powder can be added to the meal or maybe a smoothie, in which I do share some of the smoothie recipes that have helped me to build the protein in my body from time to time., just check under High Protein Smoothie Recipes.

Hemodialysis can have unpleasant side effects, (such as cramping and/or plummeting blood pressure, which is the result of fluid overload.

Peritoneal Dialysis, can lead to weight gain and a change in appearance from a bulging belly, and in some cases a patient can develop an umbilical hernia, because of the amount of dialysate being dwelled (and this could occur overtime).

ACCESS CARE:

Our access is our lifeline, and it must be properly taken care of, to assure a long life span - whether it be an AV Fistula, AV Graft or even a PD catheter. Currently I am on PD, and I know first hand, how important it is in keeping the PD catheter. My PD nurse, Tyra, taught me very well, how to care for my PD catheter, and I am aware that everyone have their own unique way of how they take care of their particular PD catheter. Let me share with you, the technique that Tyra, taught me how to care for my catheter. First, I was told to wash my hands with an antibacterial soap or sometimes I would use a waterless hand sanitizer before my catheter care. I was told to lubricate a IV gauze, with surclens (a catheter cleanser, that is supplied by Baxter, (in which I order my supplies from once a month). I would let these lubricated gauzes lay around the opening of my catheter for about 10 to 15 minutes, then I would go around in a circular motion, sometimes there is some dry blood, that may form, but the gauze lubricated with surclens, helps to loosen the dry blood, so that it can be removed with the gauze. I look at the area, after I have dried the area with the extra in used mini cap, and then I take a look at the catheter area, under and around the site, and check for drainage, or for any redness, I was told that if it does appear to be red around exit site, to call my PD nurse, and especially if I experience any pain at the exit site, but I haven't "thank God", had any issues of such, in all of my ten years so far with PD. I was also told to check for cracks, or holes in my catheter tubing. If this were to occur, I was told to place a clamp on my catheter and then call my PD nurse immediately. Also make sure after the treatment is over, and the cleansing technique is done thoroughly, then make sure to double check to make sure the transfer set is twisted well, and secure. I use silk tape to secure my transfer set and tubing. And also when I am out and about, I secure my transfer set, by a tube, (that I made from old t-shirt material, a little bit wider than the transfer set (Glo's tip: you can hand sew it real tight, if you don't own a sewing machine, I use a safety pin, to pin it to my undergarments, and this works for me, (I made several of these little transfer holders), but I only do this, when I am out and about, I usually just use silk tape when I am at home, (note: this little t-shirt technique, was created from my own personal preference), it works for me, but it may not be comfortable for other patients. You will eventually come up with your own unique way of securing your transfer set. Although you can secure your catheter simply with tape, there are other devices to help in securing your transfer set (to help keep it in place), which will keep it from being pulled or tugged in anyway, (at the exit site), which is very important to keep safe from developing an infection of such. You can ask your PD nurse at your dialysis unit, about belts of such that could be used for this purpose. I myself, prefer tape, because I have used the belt, and it is not very comfortable for me, and this is from personal preference. Always keep some slack in the catheter to avoid any tension at the exit site. My PD nurse, stressed this from time to time, during the training, that it is very important to keep the bowels moving regularly, (try not ever getting constipated), I have done pretty good with this, although, when I had to return to hemo, temporary, back in 2006, because I developed a fungus, and had to have my catheter completely removed, I began to experienced constipation, but it was a good thing that I wasn't on PD, it wasn't much of an issue with hemo, although my neph, prescribed a med, that remedied that very quickly. If you have issues with constipation, informed your PD nurse immediately about it. It is funny, when I first started PD, back in 2000, I was told that swimming was forbidden, but as the years went on, all that changed. My nephrologist said swimming is allowed, but only in a private, chlorinated pool or salt water, if recommended by your neph. Do prepare for swimming, a waterproof dressing and complete catheter care had to be done immediately after the swim. However, no hot tubs, public pools or Jacuzzi, because of the risk of possible infection development.

If you have to have an operation, while on PD, straining can cause the PD solution to have a pink color, leaks or a hernia formation can develop after a surgical procedure. After having the surgical procedure for a PD catheter, avoid straining, as straining can cause the PD solution (Dianeal), to have a pink color, and can cause leaks or hernia formation after the operation. Always life with your legs to avoid straining the abdomen and avoid heavy lifting or pushing immediately after the PD catheter has been inserted. Make sure you have the dialysis centers number and any after hour phone numbers available at all times.

CARE FOR AV GRAFT OR AV FISTULA:

* Before dialysis treatment, carefully wash the access with soap and water
* Keep your access clean and watch for swelling, redness, drainage, or tenderness in the area.
* Avoid any trauma to the access area of the graft or fistula, because injuries to the access has the potential to be life-threatening.
* Ways to keep the access from clotting
- Don't wear jewelry tight around the wrist - such as a watch, or bracelet
- Don't wear tight clothing over the access
- Don't sleep on the access
- Don't rest a purse or bag on the access area
- Avoid any heavy lifting with the access arm
- Don't allow any blood draws or blood pressure checks on the access arm
- Don't have any IV inserted on the access arm
- I used to check my access for the vibration or thrill as they use to call it, to make sure it is still functioning - like an hour before my schedule dialysis treatment and once before bedtime

- Always informed your nurse, if you notice any changes in the access vibration
- To maintain a good access, good cannulation is mandatory, but avoid cannulating the same area, especially if you have an AV Graft, I learned this the hard way, mainly because techs would not listen to me, and rotate my site, to avoid any damage to the graft. During my 10 year run with hemo, I have had my issues with techs and how they handled the cannulating of my graft, but with a fistula, you can have the buttonhole technique. Buttonholes are a wonderful way to preserve the life of the access, but a patient with a AV Graft, (like myself), aren't fortunate to use the buttonhole technique. If you have a AV Fistula, you can always ask if your particular unit offer the buttonhole technique.

I have had my issues during my 10 yr. run with hemo, when it comes to the bleeding time, when the needles are removed after treatment is completed. In 1990, when I started hemo treatment, the nurses and techs would hold the access site for you, but that changed about five years after my initial start. I noticed one day, I came in, and after the treatment was over, my tech informed me, that they weren't allowed to hold the access site for the patient, and that we were told that we had to hold our own access to stop the bleeding, or the only way they would hold it, if the patient wasn't capable of doing it for themselves. You could imagine, I wasn't very pleased with this new policy, as it freaked me out, caused I thought that I would not be able to hold the site properly, especially since the tech instructed me how to do this. I was told to apply just enough pressure to stop the bleeding, but not to stop the blood flow through the access. Then when the bleeding has stopped, place a bandage of such over the access area. Place the bandage securely, but not so tight that the patient cannot feel the thrill of the access. I know there were times, when they would secure my access, because I was known to start bleeding, even once it appears to have stopped, because I happen to be on coumadin - (a blood thinner, to prevent clotting of the access). On occasion there were times when my time spent holding my access to stop the bleeding would exceed an hour pass my scheduled time off. I was told to keep the bandage in place for a couple of hours, but there was this one time, when I had my fourth graft placed on the upper part of my left thigh, and I got home from the unit, ate lunch, and then took a nap for a couple of hours, to rejuvenate, (a routine I did on the regular three days a week after treatment), anyway I awaken from my nap, several hours after, and attempt to remove the bandage, and as soon as I removed it halfway, the blood began to shoot like a small waterfall, it was soon apparent that it was soon out of control, so of course, it was after hours, and the paramedics had to be summoned, to help in controlling it, but I won't go through the scenarios around this episode, because I have shared this in my first book "My Renal Life" (I know it, I live it). As I know, the graft or fistula access can appear hideous, don't try to hide it with tight clothing, I know in the summer, it maybe uncomfortable to wear long sleeves, to hide the access scars, but I remedied that, I just started investing in shear type blouses, which can be very comfortable in the very warm weather, just in case, you are skeptic of the appearance of your access scar or scars. Just shop around for the best bargains, they are out there, if you do the searching. All in all, following these steps, to keep your lifeline safe and most importantly a long life and infection free.

Forewords from the Author

After reading my book, I hope that you gained an insight on the dialysis life, and mostly importantly how polycystic kidney disease, develops into chronic kidney disease, which eventually will lead to end stage renal disease. The importance of getting tested for the early stages of chronic kidney disease, to start taking preventive measures to help in prolonging the onset of the development of end stage renal disease, (stage 5), but don't fret!, if your chronic kidney disease develops into end stage renal disease, you can live a long productive life with dialysis. No matter how long it takes to receive the blessing of a transplant, the disease can be managed. By educating yourself on every aspect of the management of good health with dialysis, you can maintain continued good health with dialysis.

Most important with early diagnose of polycystic kidney disease, and the possibility of chronic kidney disease, it is a known fact that high blood pressure occurs in approximately 40% of PKD patients by the time they are in their twenties (20s) and is associated with increased kidney size and left heart size, which can lead to *Congestive Heart Failure*.

To avoid cardiovascular complications, it is important for ADPKD patients to maintain their blood pressure within a normal range.

All in all, the blood pressure plays an important part in the overall health of a non-dialysis patient, as well as a patient with a dialysis life, always maintain a normal blood pressure. I share many cooking tips and home remedies to aid in the accomplishment of keeping that blood pressure in normal range, especially with this very complex renal diet, that we dialysis patients have to follow.

For over two decades, I have had my struggles off and on, with my blood pressure being in question, too elevated as well as too low at times.

BASIC HOMEMADE WHITE SAUCE
(A simple renal friendly white sauce, to enhance the flavor of many of my renal friendly recipes)

3 Tbsp. margarine
1 ½ Tbsp. cornstarch
¾ Cup Mocha Mix or Coffee Rich

Melt margarine in saucepan or over a double boiler. Remove pan from heat and cool fat until lukewarm to touch. Blend in cornstarch to make a smooth paste and add liquid slowly, stirring to blend. Cook over moderate heat for 10-15 minutes (slightly longer for double boiler), stirring occasionally. Sauce should be smooth. If it begins to boil vigorously, reduce heat.

Note: This sauce may be refrigerated and/or frozen to be used later. Simply reheat cold or frozen sauce and whisk until smooth. Add more liquid if necessary.

Glo's Tip: I use this basic white sauce in many of my renal friendly recipes, such as when I make potato clam chowder, a white sauce to pour over my chicken fried steak recipe, and a white sauce to mix in my turkey fettucine recipe. This simple to make white sauce can go a long way in many of my renal friendly recipes. I have also used this white sauce on my steamed asparagus recipe from time to time, with adding a ½ tsp. of curry powder, for a much richer robust flavor. You can also use this basic white sauce and add some sliced mushrooms to make a mushroom sauce, and also a little kitchen bouquet to bring out the color of mushroom sauce, (only a few drops, will do it for the color).

Nutritional Facts: (based on a ¼ cup serving)

Protein - 0gm   Calcium - 86mg
Sodium - 135mg   Phosphorus - 24mg
Potassium - 41mg

Check out the comparison, of making a white sauce from a mix - the advantage of making it from scratch, based on a ¼ cup serving

Protein - 2.5mg   Sodium - 200mg   Calcium - 61mg
Potassium - 111mg   Phosphorus - 64mg

OKRA CREOLE:
(consisting of Seafood, Chicken, Vegetables & Herbs)

Ingredients:

1 lb - Okra - sliced into ½ " pieces

Extra virgin olive oil) - coat the bottom of skillet

1 cup Stewed tomatoes

1 cup Roasted peppers - chopped

1 cup Green peppers - chopped

1 cup dry shrimp

½ lb - fresh shrimp - peeled

1 lb. - smoke sausage - or turkey sausage (diced)

½ lb. - boiled chicken wings

1 tsp - dry Thyme

1 tsp - dry Basil

3 bay leaves

2 ½ cup - chicken broth

1 tbsp - gumbo file

1 cup - onion, chopped

1 cup - green onions, chopped

4 clove - garlic, chopped

1 cup - celery, chopped

2 cups - long grain rice

1 cup - parsley, chopped

2 tbsp - red wine vinegar

1 tsp. - creole seasoning

1 tbsp - garlic powder

1 tbsp - onion powder

For Rice - follow package directions

Instructions:

In a skillet saute' chopped onions, peppers, garlic, celery in olive oil until vegetables are soft. Transfer vegetables to a stock pot and add the Okra, stewed tomatoes, diced sausage, boiled chicken wings, thyme, basil, bay leaf, rice wine vinegar, Creole seasoning, garlic powder, onion powder, and dry shrimp, and broth to simmer on low heat for ½ an hour, or until okra is tender, then add the shrimp, parsley and chopped green onions at the end. Remove the bay leaves Serve hot on a bed of rice. Yum Eee!

Note: To get rid of the slimy texture of the okra, add red wine vinegar.

This Okra dish is one of my favorites, because I simply love okra. I remember when my mom would make this dish, and dad wasn't a big lover of okra, he would say, you know how I like your mom to make okra, prepare it, then cook it, and dump it in the trash, boy does it taste good. I would just laugh and indulge in my okra creole.

Glo's Tip: This recipe is also great with linguine, try it you'll like it (just follow the package directions)

Nutritional Facts: (based on a ½ cup serving)

Okra has about 257 mg of potassium - (when cooked raw), and 215mg of potassium - (when cooked frozen).

Check the food finder list in this book, if you are curious about the protein, potassium and phosphorus intake of chicken, and shrimp

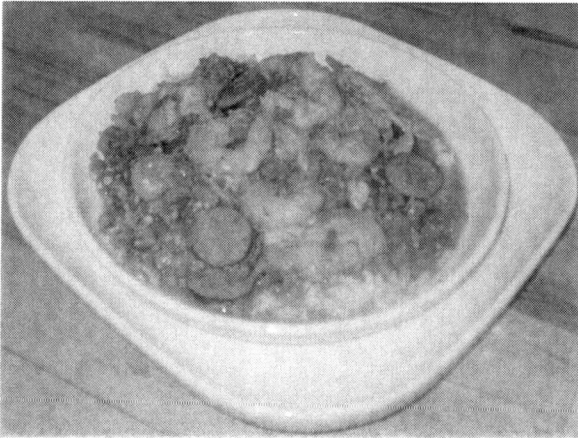

TURKEY SALAD:

Ingredients:

3 cups - cooked turkey breast (shredded or chopped if you desire)
1 ½ cup - chopped celery
¾ cup - finely chopped almonds or walnuts (watch the phosphorus, use less if necessary)
1 (one) 6 oz. Can sliced water chestnuts
A medium onion chopped
2 tsp lemon juice
1 ½ cup - mayonnaise or ranch dressing
1 - 11 oz. - can - cream of chicken soup

(SECOND GROUP OF INGREDIENTS)

¾ - cup - grated mozzarello cheese
1 ½ cup - crushed potato chips (or corn , tortilla chips, or plain cornflakes, if you prefer)

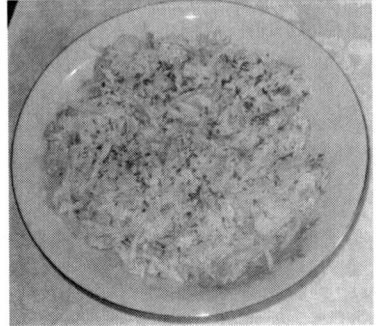

Instructions:

Mix first group of ingredients together. Place in a casserole disk and top with second group of ingredients) - Bake at 350 for 30-45 minutes until bubbly.

Glo Tip: Serve on baquettes, even great on rye bread, or if you prefer wrap the turkey salad in a butter lettuce leave - (you can also substitute to turkey breast for chicken breast, if you prefer)

A story: I landed a great job at the University of San Francisco. I attended my first potluck, And a co-worker brought in this turkey dish, and I immediately fell in love with this dish, and ask the co-worker for the recipe, and every chance I get I make this dish. Thank you Chris. Its great for little get togethers and cocktail parties also.

LUNCH TIME CROSTINI

Ingredients:

20 slices - baguettes (if diabetic - whole wheat baguette)
(½ inches thick)

1 lb. Smoked Salmon	¼ tsp - ground black pepper
1 cup - herbal cream cheese	1 tsp - garlic powder
1 English cucumber - sliced thin	½ cup - roasted red pepper (diced)
1 tsp - balsamic vinegar	1 cup - tomato - seeded & diced
1 tsp - extra virgin olive oil	1 oz. - mozzarello or provolone cheese
1 tsp - ground black pepper	1 tsp - onion powder
1 tsp - garlic salt	1 tsp - creole seasoning
1 tsp - balsamic vinegar	
1 tsp - extra virgin olive oil	
1 garlic clove - finely minced	
1 tsp - dried rosemary - crumbled	

Instructions:

Preheat the oven to 350 F. Arrange the bread slices in a single layer on a baking sheet and bake until lightly toasted, about 8 to 10 minutes.

While the bread is toasting. In a bowl, mix the vinegar, olive oil, garlic, rosemary, black pepper, garlic powder, and onion powder and stir to mix well. Then add the roasted red peppers, tomato, and cheese.

Toss gently to coat. Spoon a tablespoon of the vegetable mixture onto each toasted baguette slice.

For the Salmon Crostini: on the remainder half of the baguettes (10 ct.) - Spread a light layer of the cream cheese on each baguette, then layer a slice of smoked salmon, then place about three thin slices of cucumber and drizzle a little of the vinegar on top and sprinkle each slice of cucumber with black pepper.

Glo's tip: these baguettes are a great snack treat or as a party appetizer

I make a simple to make Peach Cobbler and I would like to share the recipe with you. It is from a recipe that I learned from a aunt of mine, way back in the 70's.

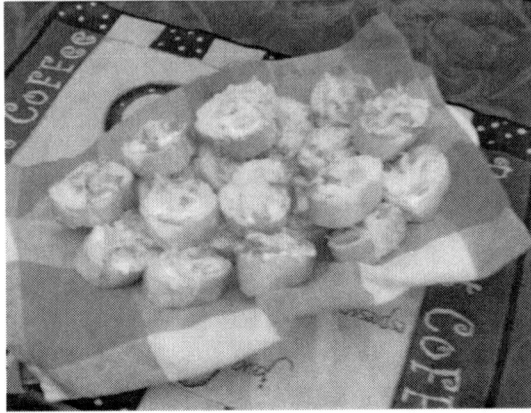

PEACH COBBLER

Peach Mixture

4 cups of fresh (peeled and sliced) or frozen sliced peaches, (if you use canned peaches, drain the liquid from them, before using) - 8 med. Size peaches is equivalent to 4 cups.

¼ cup - rum
2 cup - sugar
1 tsp - cinnamon
½ tsp - nutmeg
2 tsp - baking soda
½ tsp - salt
1 ready made pie crust

½ cup - all purpose flour
1 tbsp - brown sugar
¼ cup - margarine (melted)
1 tbsp - mocha mix
1 tsp - vanilla extract

Baking Instructions:

Preheat oven - 375 -F
In a glass casserole baking dish, add the sliced peaches, and then mix the dry ingredient in the sliced peaches first - sugar, cinnamon, flour, nutmeg, baking soda, salt brown sugar and flour. Then mix the wet ingredients in - rum, margarine, mocha mix and vanilla extract, and blend well in the peach and dry ingredient mixture.

Meanwhile, take the ready made pie crust out, to chill from the refrigerator, and then with a little flour for dusting, unroll the pie crust, and dust with a little flour, and give the crust a little bit of a roll, and then using a pizza cutter of such, cut strips to place on top of the peach mixture, in a cross over effect, as many as are needed. You know like one over, one under, and so on, until the whole peach mixture is covered, usually about six to eight strips, you can make the strips as wide as you like.

Bake at 375 for 40 to 45 minutes, until golden brown. Serve warm with whip cream or a little Ice cream (watch out for phosphorus - know your limits)

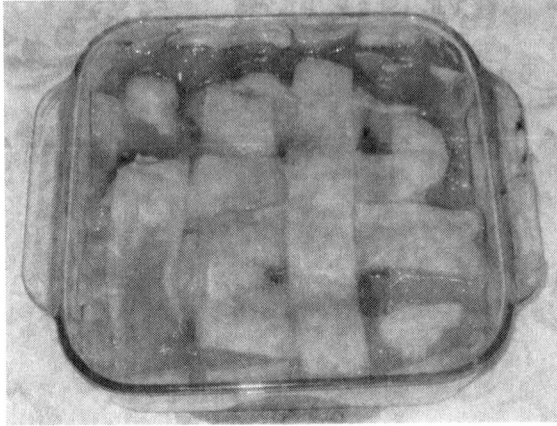

SEASONED BAKED POTATO
(Twice Baked)

Ingredients:

8 3-inch long oval-shaped
   potatoes - peeled
1 tbsp - Creole seasoning
1 ½ tbsp - Garlic powder
1 ½ tbsp - Onion powder
½ cup - grated parmesan cheese
1 cup - dry bread crumbs

4 strips of bacon, (turkey, preferably)
   - fried crispy
2 tbsp - parsley flakes
½ cup - extra virgin olive oil
½ cup - chicken broth
1 tbsp - Mrs. Dash (garlic & herb)
1 ½ cup - Mozzarello cheese

Instructions:

Preheat oven to 450 F. Cut each potato starting at one end ¼-inch slices stopping ¼-inch from bottom so slices remain attached. Place potatoes with sliced edges upward into a well greased shallow baking dish. Then brush a light coating of olive oil on each potato, place chicken broth on bottom of baking dish, and place in oven. Bake in oven for 30 minutes, basting occasionally with olive oil & chicken broth mixture in pan.

Take the potatoes out of the oven, and cool, then remove the filling of each potato, and place in a bowl, and Sprinkle with Creole seasoning, onion & garlic powder, herb Mrs. Dash, parsley flakes, mix the seasoning mixture into the potato filling, and crumble bacon to add to the seasoning mixture and blend well.

Mix cheese and bread crumbs; sprinkle over the top of each potato, then sprinkle some shredded mozzarello cheese on top. Bake another 30 minutes without basting, or until the potatoes are golden brown and tender.

Glo's Tip - Being a dialysis patient, you need to soak your potatoes over night (look back at the topic on leeching) or about six hours, to get rid of some of the starch - (where most of the potassium lies) But there is no need, if at the time you may not have any issues with your potassium, but make sure wish applies to you.

You can substitute the mozzarello cheese for any type of cheese you want, but be wised to the amount of phosphorus a cheese contains, (check back at the phosphorus chart finder for the contents of various cheeses)

Nutrition Facts:

One (1) large potato - no skin - 610 mg, but a large potato with the skin is 844 mg, calorie - 138, carbohydrates - 24g, Protein - 2g, fat - 4g, fiber - 4g, cholesterol - 6mg, sodium - 89mg

Note: FYI: phosphorus - one large potato, baked - without skin - is equivalent to 610mg of phosphorus

One large potato, baked - with skin - 844mg of phosphorus

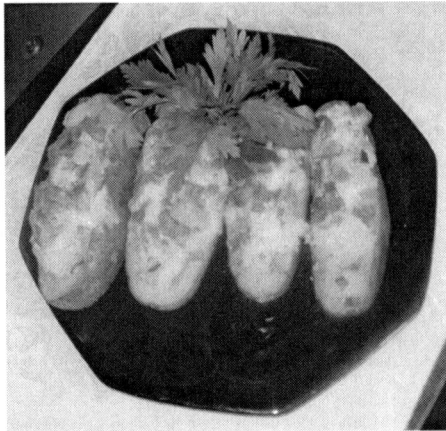

FRIED ZUCCHINI

Ingredients:

3 or 4 Medium Zucchini, cut,
   (cut in ½ in. slices)
1 cup - milk or mocha mix
1 cup - flour
¼ cup - grated parmesan cheese
1 tsp - dry basil leaves
½ tsp - thyme

½ tsp - tarragon
½ tsp - creole seasoning
½ tbsp - onion & garlic powder
½ tsp - black pepper
flavored breadcrumbs - shrimp or Italian
2 ½ tbsp - canola oil

Instructions:

Season Zucchini slices with creole seasoning, onion & garlic powder, set aside. And then setup up three pans for dipping - one for flour parmesan, basil, thyme, tarragon and pepper mixture, milk & egg mixture, and bread crumb mixture. Start dipping the zucchini sticks one by one in each of the dipping pans and heat oil and fry. Serve hot.

Glo' tip: You can also substitute the zucchini, for eggplant, or make an assortment of both vegetables

FYI: There is about 100 mg of phosphorus in this dish, if you use milk instead of using mocha mix. From the chart finder, the potassium in this dish is high, (about 245 mg) so please I can't stress this enough, take your binders, and if you eat slow, like I do, take half your binders at the beginning of your meal, and take the rest in the middle or at the very end of your meal. (they will work better, trust me).

If you can't found shrimp flavored breadcrumbs - purchase some dry shrimps - and make breadcrumbs with a food processor, you can add a little Italian seasonings to the shrimp breadcrumbs for more flavor

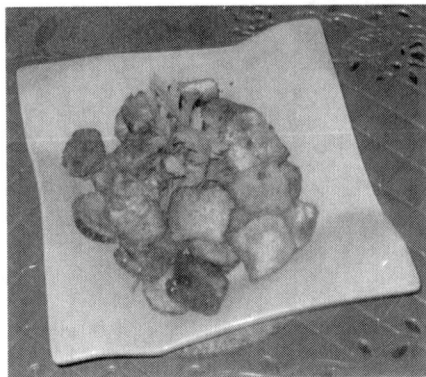

Ending Thoughts

My motto has always been "Don't let kidney disease control you" "You control the disease and even if you have pain that you think you can't bare, just remember you will never suffer as much as our Lord and Savoir, Jesus Christ did.

Index

To all my readers: This second book has black and white images of various renal friendly recipes, which was a part of my publishing package deal, but I am going to publish a second book, in a few months, with color images of my recipes, and the third book will mainly be a renal cookbook, and keep in mind, I am a non-diabetic dialysis patient. In this second book, I just thought I would share some of my recipes with images, so you could see what the finish product (recipe), would look like, even though it is in black and white, so don't get discouraged, the most important thing about this book, is that I am revealing my dialysis experience and history, which is more beneficial than recipes, but of course, recipes will help you to get a better grasp and understanding of this very complex renal diet.

CPSIA information can be obtained
at www.ICGtesting.com
Printed in the USA
LVOW11s1258170417
531091LV00001B/76/P